はじめての薬学英語

野口ジュディー／神前陽子／スミス朋子／天ヶ瀬葉子［著］

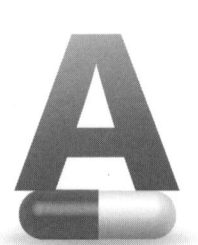
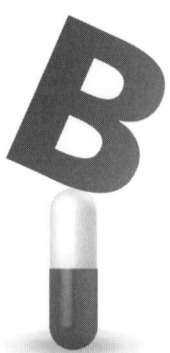
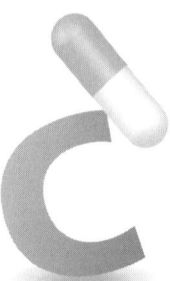

First Steps in English
for
Pharmaceutical
Sciences

講談社

あらかじめご了承ください

・本書は全国の大学・専門学校で教材として使用されているため、練習問題の解答や日本語訳は付属していません。

まえがき

　今日、英語が医療分野のlingua franca（国際共通言語）になっていることへの対応として、薬学英語の充実を図ることの重要性が指摘されています。しかし、薬学英語を低学年から導入している薬学部・薬科大学はまだまだ少ないのが現状です。読む・聞く・話す・書くというスキルを総合的に扱いながら、1年生からでも薬学英語の指導はできると私たちは考えています。

　では、初めて出会う薬学英語として、何をどのように学べばいいのでしょうか？　この問いに対する答えを探しながら、英語教師、薬剤師・薬学研究者と薬学生が知恵を結集して、「はじめての薬学英語」を上梓しました。薬学生には、専門英語の授業でどのようなことに興味を感じ、また学びたいかを尋ねました。将来、役に立つものを学びたいということと、オーセンティックな文書（英語教育用に作成されたものではなく、「本物」の文書）に触れるとモチベーションが上がるといったコメントが印象的でした。薬剤師・薬学研究者らは自らの海外経験（イギリスとアメリカ）から必要な種類（ジャンル）の文書を提案し、英語教師らは長年、薬学生に専門英語を教えてきた経験にもとづいて文書への取り組み方を検討しました。

　このアプローチはESP（English for Specific Purposes）専門英語教育の理論に基づいています。特定の分野で専門言語を駆使している専門家から情報を得て、分野で仕事をする際に必要なことがらを効率よく学ぶ方法です。ESPでは、単なる専門用語だけでなく、使用される文書の種類（ジャンル）と、それによって決定される情報のフレームワーク（情報の提示される順序と論理）も重視します。この教科書に掲載されている様々な文書は、すべて薬学関係のものであり、それぞれに特定の目的（purpose）と想定する読者（audience）を明確に持ち、かなりの部分定型化された伝えるべき情報（information）を含みます。みなさんが勉強するのは、このようなはっきりした目的を持った文書の言語的特徴（language features）です。この四つの要素の頭文字を取ってPAIL（バケツという意味の英単語）、つまり、文書のメッセージに対する内容物の「入れ物」について学ぶのだと考えるとわかりやすいでしょう。

　この本の執筆にあたって、貴重な情報を提供してくださった薬学部の学生のみなさん、現在アメリカで薬剤師として活躍されているDr. Mariko Ono Guest、イギリスのカーディフ大学薬学部Dr. Robert D. E. Sewell、そして、終始適切なサポートを賜った講談社サイエンティフィクの小笠原弘高氏に深く感謝いたします。

著者一同

CONTENTS

まえがき iii

Unit 1 アドバイス情報：子供の良い食習慣作り（一般向け）............ 1
Healthy Eating
　　Relaxing a bit　ウェブでレシピを検索 8

Unit 2 職務記述：薬剤師の職務（英語学習者向けのニュース番組）...... 9
What It Takes to Become a Druggist
　　Relaxing a bit　日米英の薬剤師の資格の比較 16

Unit 3 商品説明：サプリメントについて（一般向け）...................... 18
Coenzyme Q-10
　　Relaxing a bit　ハーブや薬草の名前 25

Unit 4 薬の箱：医薬品情報（一般向け）.. 26
Paracetamol + Codeine + Caffeine Combination
　　Relaxing a bit　元素や化合物の読み方 37

Unit 5 新聞コラム：薬の飲み方について（一般向け）...................... 38
To Your Health / A spoonful of sugar makes the medicine go down
　　Relaxing a bit　医療に関する文化の違い 44

Unit 6 教科書：心臓について（高校生向け）.................................... 45
The Mammalian Heart
　　Relaxing a bit　科学英語の複数形：ラテン語・ギリシャ語から 53

Unit 7 健康勧告：サルモネラ菌から身を守る（一般向け）................ 54
Be Salmonella Safe!
　　Relaxing a bit　数字の読み方 63

Unit 8 疾患情報：肝炎（一般向け）.. 64
Hepatitis C Information for the Public
　　Relaxing a bit　ウイルスの発見 76

Unit 9 法律・規制情報：化粧品と医薬品の違い（一般向け）............ 77
Is It a Cosmetic, a Drug, or Both? (Or Is It Soap?)
　　Relaxing a bit　法律関係の文書名の読み方 88

Unit 10 医学系学術誌の記事：不思議な猫の話（学術誌の購読者向け）...... 89
A Day in the Life of Oscar the Cat
　　Relaxing a bit　学術論文のオープンアクセス化 99

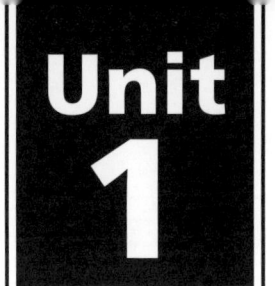

Examining the source

　NHS (National Health Service) は、税金と社会保険料を財源としたイギリスの国営医療制度で、イギリスに居住する人はNHSによる医療を無料で受けられます。また、調剤薬局で患者が処方薬に支払う金額はどの薬でも一律の価格になっています。NHSでは処方権を持った薬剤師が患者に直接処方し投薬することもあります。さらに、ウェブサイト (http://www.nhs.uk/Pages/HomePage.aspxなど) から、市民向けの医療や健康維持に関する情報をイラストやビデオを使って発信しています。Unit 1では、http://www.northsomerset.nhs.uk/ よりその１つを取りあげます。

Getting to know the genre

テキストを詳しく読む前に次の1〜5に答えましょう。
Take a look at the text and answer the following questions.

1. What do you think this text is?

2. What is the purpose of this text?

3. Who is the audience for this text?

4. What kind of information does it give?

5. What are the language features of this text?

Reading the text → CD Track 01

NHS
North Somerset

Healthy Eating

Top tips for top kids!

We all want our children to grow up to be happy, healthy adults. But it can sometimes be hard to know how. So here are 6 easy tips to help you keep your kids feeling great. These tips have been put together by health professionals and will help your kids to eat well, move more and live longer.

Whatever their weight, it's important that children eat properly and get lots of exercise to build a healthy body. If they're carrying too much fat in their bodies, they are at a greater risk of heart disease and diabetes in later life. If they're underweight it's just as important for them to eat healthy food and be active. If you ever have any concerns about your kids' health or weight – please contact your GP.

Top tip 1

Sugar swaps

Swapping sugary snacks and drinks for ones that are lower in sugar can make a huge difference to kids' calorie intake.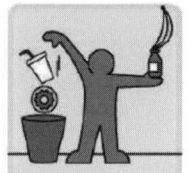
Not only that, but it's better for their teeth too.

Top tip 2
Meal time

It's important for kids to have regular, proper meals as growing bodies respond better to routine.

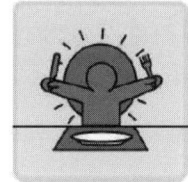

Top tip 3
Me size meals

Even though they're growing, it's important to make sure kids get just the right amount for their age – not too little and not too much.

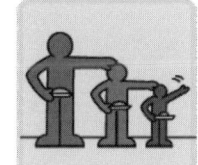

Top tip 4
Snack check

Many snacks are full of the things that are bad for us – sugar, salt, fat and calories. So try and keep a careful eye on how many the kids are having.

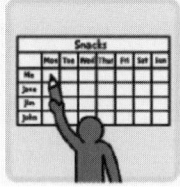

Top tip 5
5 A DAY

It's easier than you think to give your kids five portions of fruit and vegetables a day. For kids, one portion is roughly a handful.

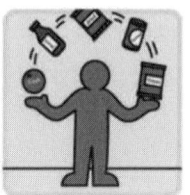

Top tip 6
Cut back fat

We all know too much fat is bad for us. But it's not always easy to tell where it's lurking.

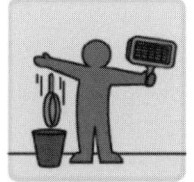

Note

Note: 5 a dayは、1日400gの野菜や果物を摂取すると、脳・心臓の疾患や肥満・2型糖尿病のリスクを下げるということでWHO世界保健機関が推奨しているもので、いくつかの国でキャンペーンが行われています。One portionは80gで野菜（じゃがいもを除く）や果物の中から5種類のものを選んで食べましょう、というものです。

2021年6月現在、NHSのLibraryからPDFをダウンロードできます。
https://www.lnds.nhs.uk/Library/change4lifetopstipsforkidsdh_093121.pdf

❶ Checking the terms

GLOSSARY

diabetes	糖尿病	portion	食事などの一人分の量
GP	ホームドクター、かかりつけの総合診療医 (general practitioner)	routine	習慣、日課
intake	摂取	swap ~ for	~を…と交換する
lurk	[危険などが] 潜む		

 Learning the vocabulary

以下は覚えておくと便利な表現です。最適なものを選んで、1〜10の文を完成させましょう。
Here are some phrases that are useful to know. Choose the best phrase to complete each sentence below.

60 minutes worth of	put together
a greater risk of	sit still
burn off	the right amount for
keep an eye on	underweight
proper meal	worn out

1. You need to eat a (1)_____ in the morning to be alert in school.
2. The child is (2)_____ for his age.
3. Kids should get at least (3)_____ exercise a day to keep healthy.
4. There is (4)_____ suffering from disease if you do not eat well.
5. Exercise can (5)_____ excessive fat.

4

6. She (6)_____ a lunchbox for him to take to the picnic.

7. The mother was (7)_____ from caring all night for the sick child.

8. (8)_____ the young child to prevent him from getting hurt.

9. You should know (9)_____ you if you wish to keep health.

10. Please (10)_____ for the group photograph.

Understanding the material

以下の1〜8の説明文はTop Tip 1〜6のどの内容に対応しますか？
Match the following with the Top Tip in the reading section.

1. Try to organise the day around three regular mealtimes – it's easier to keep kids from pestering for snacks if they know when their next meal is coming!　　(No.　　)

2. Keep count. Many people are surprised when they actually count up how many sweets, crisps, and biscuits they get through. Keep count and you're more likely to cut down – which is good for your kids and for your purse too.
(No.　　)

3. Swap to water, semi-skimmed milk (but remember children under 2 need full-fat milk) or diluted fresh fruit juice instead of drinks with added sugar like cola or squash.
(No.　　)

4. Remember that kids are smaller than adults. It sounds obvious, but an adult tummy is much bigger than a kid's tummy – so try and give them a portion that matches their size and not the same amount of food as you.

(No.   )

5. Don't forget that it is sometimes kinder to say no. We all love to give our kids what they want, but try to find different ways to reward them – stickers, or a trip to the park.

(No.   )

6. Get them to drink a portion. One glass of unsweetened fruit juice or one smoothie a day count as one of the five.

(No.   )

7. Literally cut the fat. Trim off any fat you can see from meat before you cook it, and skin chicken and turkey first. Draining off the fat after cooking will also help.

(No.   )

8. Frozen and canned fruit and vegetables count too. It's quick and cheap to boil some frozen peas or open a can of sweetcorn.

(No.   )

Trying out the genre

次のリストから最適な単語を選んで(1)～(10)に入れ、文を完成させましょう。また、本文のTop Tip 1～6のどの内容と対応するか答えましょう。

Complete the following sentences with the best choice from the following list. After doing that, decide which Top Tip the item matches.

| copy | eat | grilling | piece | try |
| designed | frying | instead | switch | watch |

1. (1)_____ packaging sizes. Lots of foods and drinks, like cans of pop, are (2)_____ for adults or for sharing. (No.   )

2. (3)_____ to snacks like fresh or dried fruit, breadsticks and unsalted nuts (4)_____ of sweets or biscuits. (No.   )

3. A (5)_____ of fruit or vegetable can help cheer up a lunchbox. (6)_____ carrot sticks, baby tomatoes or a banana with a face drawn on the skin. (No.   )

4. (7)_____ or baking food in the oven rather than (8)_____ it on the cooker can reduce the fat content by as much as two-thirds. (No.   )

5. (9)_____ together whenever you can. Kids (10)_____ parents, brothers, sisters and friends – so when they see other people happily eating lots of different, healthy foods, they'll follow suit. (No.   )

Applying what you learned

テキストのような健康に関するadvisory sheet（アドバイス記事）を作成してみましょう。最初に以下の項目を決めて、取り掛かりましょう。

Prepare an advisory sheet. First, decide on the following:

Title

Purpose

Audience

Information to include

 Relaxing a bit

　　インターネットでお気に入りのレシピを探してみましょう。

ブルーベリーパンケーキのレシピです。

https://kidshealth.org/en/parents/blueberry-pancakes.html?WT.ac=ctg#catrecipes-family

たったの５分で作れるヘルシーなスムージー！

https://kidshealth.org/en/teens/strawberry-smoothie.html?WT.ac=ctg

音声読み上げが可能です！

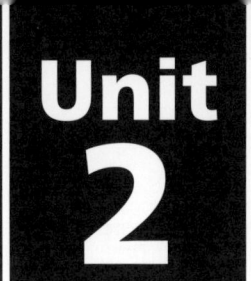

Examining the source

このUnitのテキスト「VOA Special English」は、VOA (Voice of America)が1959年から世界中の英語学習者に向けて発信している英語のニュース番組です。現在では、この番組はネット上で字幕付き音声ビデオとして提供されています。初級上から中級レベルの学習者を対象としており、単語レベルや発話のスピードもこのレベルに合わせています。

Getting to know the genre

テキストを詳しく読む前に次の1〜5に答えましょう。
Take a look at the text and answer the following questions.

1. What do you think this text is?

2. What is the purpose of this text?

3. Who is the audience for this text?

4. What kind of information does it give?

5. What are the language features of this text?

Reading the text → CD Track 02

What It Takes to Become a Druggist

BOB DOUGHTY: A listener in Vietnam wrote to thank us for the recent program about how to become a doctor in the United States. Kim Anh Nguyen was wondering if we also could explain the process of becoming a pharmacist.

We suspect the abilities needed for a career in pharmacy are about the same worldwide. They include excellent skills in science and mathematics, and the ability to communicate and work well with people.

The United States Bureau of Labor Statistics also suggests that a pharmacist needs to have good feet! Many pharmacists stand all day at work.

SHIRLEY GRIFFITH: There were almost two hundred seventy thousand pharmacists in the United States in two thousand eight. That is the most recent year for which numbers are available.

In some parts of the country, the average yearly pay for a pharmacist was almost one hundred thousand dollars. Many pharmacists work forty hours a week. But some have longer workdays. And some jobs require working at night or on weekends and holidays.

BOB DOUGHTY: A pharmacist in America is often called a druggist. Many druggists work in community pharmacies or food stores. They provide patients with prescription medicines from their doctors. Pharmacists guide patients in how to take these drugs.

Many pharmacists advise people about general health issues, like diet or exercise. Pharmacists help patients guard against dangerous drug reactions by keeping records of the drugs ordered for them by several doctors.

Pharmacists in hospitals prepare medicines and advise doctors on the choice and effects of drugs. They also plan and watch over patients' drug regimens - the systematic plans for how medicine is to be administered.

Druggists who own or operate pharmacies may sell other, non-medicinal products. They also may offer employment to and supervise other workers in the store.

Other pharmacists do research in pharmacology colleges. Some work for drug or insurance companies.

SHIRLEY GRIFFITH: A man or woman who wants to be a pharmacist needs at least six years of study on the college and college-graduate level. Some pharmacists study for eight or more years.

People who want a career as a pharmacist need to plan ahead. It is a good idea to study science in high school. Colleges and universities that have pharmacy schools require college courses in science.

Most people seeking to enter pharmacy schools attend two years or more of college. During that time they take classes in subjects including natural sciences, mathematics and biology. They also study social science and humanities like languages, history and philosophy.

BOB DOUGHTY: Someone who gains admission and completes pharmacy school earns a doctor's degree in pharmacy, called a Pharm. D. But even after the study program is completed, people cannot work as pharmacists until they take examinations to receive a license or permit.

The Department of Labor says all fifty states and Guam, Puerto Rico and the American Virgin Islands require this document.

Voice of America, 11/13/2011より

Checking the terms

GLOSSARY

administer	[薬などを]投与する	issue	関心事、大切なこと
available	入手できる	pharmacist	薬剤師
community pharmacy	地域薬局 ※hospital pharmacy＝病院薬局	pharmacy	薬学
		plan ahead	前もって計画する
drug regimen	投薬計画 ※症状に応じた薬の種類、量や回数	prescription	処方、処方箋
earn a degree	学位を取る	require	～を必要とする、求める
guard against	～を防ぐ	seek	～しようとする(試みる・努める)
have longer workdays	就労日の労働時間が長い	supervise	[仕事をする人や組織を]監督する
		suspect	～だろうと思う
humanities	人文学	watch over	～の世話をする、管理する
insurance	保険		

Learning the vocabulary

動詞の使われ方に注目しましょう。1～8とA～Hを結びつけてセンテンスを完成させましょう。
Observe how the verbs are used in the text. Match the sentence start with the best ending.

1	After passing the entrance exam, he gained	A	a degree in medicine.
2	She passed the exams and received	B	a license to practice pharmacy.
3	The nurse watched	C	admission to the university.
4	He wants to do research	D	on cancer drugs.
5	She works	E	over the patient's diet regimen.
6	The doctor advised	F	the patient about the treatment choices.
7	He studied hard to earn	G	the patient with the medicine.
8	The pharmacist provided	H	well with people.

Understanding the material

次の1〜5にセンテンスの形で答えましょう。
Answer the following questions with complete sentences.

1. What kinds of skills should a person have if he or she wants to become a pharmacist?

2. About how much does a pharmacist receive a year in the United States? How much would that be in Japanese yen at the current rate?

3. What are pharmacists called in the United States?

4. What do pharmacists who work in hospitals do in the United States?

5. If a person wants to become a pharmacist, what should he or she do?

Trying out the genre

医師助手の仕事についての説明文を読み、CDを聴いて、後のTranscriptの空所をうめましょう。完成したTranscriptを、実際にレポートするようなつもりで音読してみましょう。　→ CD Track 03

Complete the following transcript about the work of a physician assistant based on the information provided. Read it aloud as though you were the reporter.

What Physician Assistants Do

Physician assistants, also known as PAs, practice medicine under the direction of physicians and surgeons. They are formally trained to examine patients, diagnose injuries and illnesses, and provide treatment.

Work Environment

Physician assistants work in physicians' offices, hospitals, and other healthcare settings. Most work full time.

How to Become a Physician Assistant

Most physician assistants have a bachelor's degree. Then, they must complete an accredited educational program for physician assistants. That usually takes at least 2 years of full-time study and typically leads to a master's degree. All states require physician assistants be licensed.

Pay

The median annual wage of physician assistants was $86,410 in May 2010.

U. S. Bureau of Labor Statistics, OCCUPATIONAL OUTLOOK HANDBOOK より

Transcript

以下のa～hから適切なものを選んで空欄(1)～(8)に入れてTranscriptを完成させましょう。そのあと、アナウンサーのように読みあげましょう。

Complete the transcript with the choices from a to h. Read it aloud as though you were the anonouncer.

a. $86,410
b. 2010
c. a bachelor's degree
d. an accredited educational program
e. physicians' offices, hospitals, and other healthcare settings
f. to receive a license
g. two years of study
h. under the direction of physicians and surgeons

There were about 83,600 physician assistants in the United States in (1)_____ and the average yearly pay was (2)_____. Physician assistants work in (3)_____ They examine patients, diagnose injuries and illnesses and provide treatment (4)_____. A person who wants to be a physician assistant needs to have (5)_____ and complete (6)_____ for physician assistants. This requires (7)_____ and usually leads to a master's degree. People cannot work as physician assistants until they take examinations (8)_____.

→ CD Track 04

Applying what you learned

アメリカ合衆国労働省労働統計局のホームページ(http://www.bls.gov/ooh/)で、興味のある薬学関連の職業についての紹介文を読み、その内容を発表してみましょう。

Go to the Occupational Outlook Handbook of the Bureau of Labor Statistics website (http://www.bls.gov/ooh/) and find an occupation to describe using the transcript format given above.

Relaxing a bit

日本、アメリカ、イギリスの薬学教育と薬剤師を比較してみましょう。

	日本	アメリカ	イギリス
よび方	薬剤師	Pharmacist, Druggist	Pharmacist, Chemist, Druggist
薬学部入学条件	高校卒業以上	大学卒業以上	高校卒業以上
修業年限など	6年間(実務実習を含む)	*4年間(実務実習を含む)	**4年間+1年間の実務実習
取得できる学位	薬学士	Pharm.D. (Doctor of Pharmacy)	M.Pharm. (Master of Pharmacy)
国家試験について	卒業後すぐ受験可 年1回 受験回数制限なし	卒業後すぐ受験可 専門科目と薬事法の2種類の試験 一定期間後再受験可 テストセンターが開いている限りいつでも受験可	卒業後1年間の実務実習(有給)修了後に受験可 試験は夏と秋の年2回 受験回数制限3回まで
薬剤師のレベル(職位)や種類	認定薬剤師 専門薬剤師 指導薬剤師 各学会や職能団体による認定 とくにレベルはない	各種専門薬剤師 • Ambulatory care pharmacist • Critical care pharmacist • Nuclear pharmacist • Pharmacotherapy pharmacist 他がある 薬剤師として規定の経験を積んだうえでBoard of Pharmacy Specialtiesの試験に合格することで認定 レベルはない	• Pharmacist entry level • Pharmacist • Pharmacist specialist • Pharmacist advanced • Pharmacist team manager • Pharmacist consultant • Professional manager pharmaceutical services NHS (National Health Service)によるhospital pharmacistの7段階レベル

* 大学院レベルでの教育なので学位はdoctor's degree(博士号)を取得します。

** 学部レベルでの教育ですが、他学部が3年間でbachelor's degree(学士号)を取るのに対し、4年間の教育を受けるため、master's degree(修士号)を取得します。

日本、アメリカ、イギリスの薬剤師をサポートする職種について比較してみましょう。

	日本	アメリカ	イギリス
薬剤師をサポートする職種	登録販売者 調剤助手	Pharmacy technician	Pharmacy technician
専門学校入学条件	高校卒業以上	高校卒業か同等	高校卒業か同等
資格を取得する為の条件や専門学校について	専門学校は必須ではないが登録販売者は資格試験受験条件に実務経験が必要	専門学校で学ぶか、薬局で実地で学ぶ	2年間薬局で実務実習を受けながら専門学校に通う
資格	登録販売者は都道府県認定資格	統一国家資格は無いが、各専門学校が修了証や認定証などを発行 必ずしも資格は必要ではない	統一国家資格は無いが、各専門学校が修了証や認定証などを発行
レベル（職位）や種類	とくになし	店や会社の規定でレベルがあり、レベルにより任される仕事内容が違う	• Pharmacy technician • Pharmacy technician specialist • Pharmacy technician team manager NHS (National Health Service)によるhospital pharmacy technicianの3段階レベルでレベルにより任される仕事内容が違う

下記も参照してみましょう。

アメリカの薬剤師国家試験について

National Association of Boards of Pharmacy (https://nabp.pharmacy)

アメリカの専門薬剤師の仕事について

Board of Pharmacy Specialties (http://www.bpsweb.org)

イギリスの薬剤師国家試験について

General Pharmaceutical Council (http://www.pharmacyregulation.org/)

イギリスの薬剤師の仕事について

Royal Pharmaceutical Society /Careers information (https://www.rpharms.com/pharmacycareers)

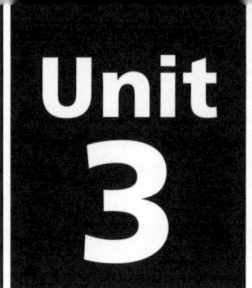

Examining the source

　MedlinePlus は National Institutes of Health（国立衛生研究所）が提供する患者やその家族や友人たちのための信頼できるウェブサイトです。病気とその状況に関する最新情報がわかりやすく説明されているのは、National Library of Medicine（アメリカ国立医学図書館）が作成しているページです。また、Drugs & Supplements のページでは、薬とサプリメントの情報がアルファベット順に提供されています。

Getting to know the genre

テキストを詳しく読む前に次の1〜5に答えましょう。
Take a look at the text and answer to the following questions.

1. What do you think this text is?

2. What is the purpose of this text?

3. Who is the audience for this text?

4. What kind of information does it give?

5. What are the language features of this text?

Reading the text → CD Track 05

Coenzyme Q-10

What is it?

Coenzyme Q-10 (CoQ-10) is a vitamin-like substance found throughout the body, but especially in the heart, liver, kidney, and pancreas. It is eaten in small amounts in meats and seafood. Coenzyme Q-10 can also be made in a laboratory. It is used as medicine.

Many people use coenzyme Q-10 for treating heart and blood vessel conditions such as congestive heart failure (CHF), chest pain (angina), high blood pressure, and heart problems linked to certain cancer drugs. It is also used for diabetes, gum disease (both taken by mouth and applied directly to the gums), breast cancer, Huntington's disease, Parkinson's disease, muscular dystrophy, increasing exercise tolerance, chronic fatigue syndrome (CFS), and Lyme disease. Some people think coenzyme Q-10 will treat hair loss related to taking warfarin (Coumadin), a medication used to slow blood clotting.

Some people also think coenzyme Q-10 might help increase energy. This is because coenzyme Q-10 has a role in producing ATP, a molecule in body cells that functions like a rechargeable battery in the transfer of energy. Coenzyme Q-10 has been tried for treating inherited or acquired disorders that limit energy production in the cells of the body (mitochondrial disorders), and for improving exercise performance.

Some people have also used coenzyme Q-10 for strengthening the immune systems of people with HIV/AIDS, male infertility, migraine headache, and counteracting muscle pain sometimes caused by a group of cholesterol-lowering medications called "statins."

Coenzyme Q-10 has even been tried for increasing life span. This idea got started because coenzyme Q-10 levels are highest in the first 20 years of life. By age 80, coenzyme-Q10 levels can be lower than they were at birth. Some people thought that restoring high levels of coenzyme-Q10 late in life might cause people to live longer. The idea works in bacteria, but not in lab rats. More research is needed to see if this works in people.

It's not only time that uses up the body's store of coenzyme Q-10. Smoking does, too.

Coenzyme Q-10 was first identified in 1957. The "Q-10" refers to the chemical make-up of the substance. These days coenzyme Q-10 is used by millions of people in Japan for heart disease, especially congestive heart failure. Coenzyme Q-10 is also used extensively in Europe and Russia. Most of the coenzyme Q-10 used in the US and Canada is supplied by Japanese companies. Coenzyme Q-10 is manufactured by fermenting beets and sugar cane with special strains of yeast.

How does it work?
Coenzyme Q-10 is an important vitamin-like substance required for the proper function of many organs and

chemical reactions in the body. It helps provide energy to cells. Coenzyme Q-10 also seems to have antioxidant activity. People with certain diseases, such as congestive heart failure, high blood pressure, periodontal disease, Parkinson's disease, certain muscular diseases, and AIDS, might have lower levels of coenzyme Q-10.

Excerpted with permission from Natural Medicines, Comprehensive Database, www..naturaldatabase, accessed 10/21/2011 より
（2012年8月MedlinePlus掲載）

Checking the terms

GLOSSARY

angina	狭心症	linked to	～と関係（関連）がある（している）
antioxidant	酸化防止剤	Lyme disease	ライム病 ※マダニによって媒介される、細菌による人獣共通感染症
blood clotting	血液凝固	male infertility	男性不妊
breast cancer	乳癌	migraine headache	片頭痛
chronic fatigue syndrome	慢性疲労症候群	mitochondrial disorders	ミトコンドリア異常
coenzyme	コエンザイム、補酵素	molecule	分子
congestive heart failure	うっ血[性]心不全	muscular dystrophy	筋ジストロフィー
counteracting	対抗[対処]するための	pancreas	膵臓
diabetes	糖尿病	Parkinson's disease	パーキンソン病
exercise tolerance	運動耐容能	periodontal	歯周の
fermenting	発酵、発酵の	statins	スタチン類 ※抗脂血症薬の一群
gum disease	歯周病、歯肉疾患	warfarin	ワルファリン ※抗血栓薬の一種
Huntington's disease	ハンチントン病		
life span	寿命、生存期間		

Learning the vocabulary

次のリストの単語およびフレーズから最も適当なものを選び、必要なら形を変えて1～10のセンテンスを完成させましょう。

Complete the following sentences with the best choice from the following list of terms.

acquired disorder	congestive heart failure
angina	inherited disorder
antioxidant activity	migraine headache
chronic fatigue syndrome	muscular dystrophy
coenzyme	periodontal disease

1. A (1)_____ seems to be caused by the actions of certain chemicals in the brain.
2. (2)_____ prevents the oxidation of compounds to reduce the amount of free radicals.
3. In (3)_____, the musculoskeletal system weakens and a person loses the ability to move.
4. A (4)_____ is an organic molecule that helps an enzyme carry out its work.
5. AIDS is an (5)_____ that occurs after birth.
6. After feeling very tired for a long time, she was diagnosed as having (6)_____.
7. In (7)_____, the heart cannot effectively pump blood.
8. An (8)_____ is genetically passed from parent to child.
9. (9)_____ is chest pain that occurs due to insufficient oxygen supply to the heart muscles.
10. In (10)_____, bacteria attack the gums, which can lead to loss of teeth.

Understanding the material

テキストはインターネット文書の抜粋です。オリジナルの文書にはこの本文のほかに5つのセクションがあります。セクション・ヘディングからそれぞれのセクションに含まれる内容を類推して結びつけてみましょう。とくに、下線の引かれている部分に注目してください。

This text has much more information that presented above. Here are five other sections that appear on the website. Match the information given below with the heading of the section. Use the underlined hint expressions to help you classify the information.

セクション・ヘディング / 含まれる内容

1. How effective is it?   (   )
2. Are there safety concerns?   (   )
3. Are there interactions with medications?   (   )
4. Are there interactions with herbs and supplements?   (   )
5. What dose is used?   (   )

セクションに含まれている内容

A. For high blood pressure: 120-200 mg per day divided into 2 doses.

B. Taking coenzyme Q-10 does not seem to decrease high cholesterol or triglycerides.

C. Warfarin (Coumadin) is used to slow blood clotting while coenzyme Q-10 might increase blood clotting.

D. Coenzyme Q-10 is POSSIBLY SAFE for children. But coenzyme Q-10 should not be used in children without medical supervision.

E. Taking coenzyme Q-10 also appears to reduce migraine frequency in children who have low levels of coenzyme Q-10.

F. For reducing the risk of future cardiac events in patients with recent myocardial infarction: 120 mg daily in 2 divided doses.

G. While most people tolerate coenzyme Q-10 well, it can cause some mild side effects including stomach upset, loss of appetite, nausea, vomiting, and diarrhea. It can cause allergic skin rashes in some people.

H. Taking a combination of coenzyme Q-10, berberine, policosanol, red yeast rice, folic acid and astaxanthin reduces cholesterol levels.

I. There is conflicting research about the effectiveness of coenzyme Q-10 for diabetes. Some research shows that taking coenzyme Q-10 might lower blood sugar levels. But other research has found no benefit.

Trying out the genre

アロエに関する記述です。順不同に並んでいるセンテンスを、正しく並び替えて意味の通る文にしましょう。

Here are sentences from a description of Aloe from the same website. Arrange them in the best order for the explanation.

1. A number of years ago, the FDA became concerned about the safety of aloe latex, which was an ingredient in many laxatives.
2. Aloe medications can be taken by mouth or applied to the skin.
3. Some people take aloe latex by mouth, usually for constipation.
4. Aloe (often called aloe vera) is a plant related to cactus.
5. The FDA's concern was heightened by the fact that people develop a kind of "tolerance" to aloe latex.
6. But most people use aloe gel topically, as a remedy for skin conditions including burns, sunburn, frostbite, psoriasis, and cold sores.
7. Aloe gel is taken by mouth for osteoarthritis, bowel diseases including ulcerative colitis, fever, itching and inflammation, and as a general tonic.
8. It produces two substances, gel and latex, which are used for medicines.

(　　) → (　　) → (　　) → (　　) → (　　)
→ (　　) → (　　) → (　　)

📋 Applying what you learned

MedlinePlus Herbs and Supplements Website で、知っている植物、ハーブ類（bilberry, blueberry, black tea, green tea など）や物質（calcium, magnesium, vitamin など）を調べてみましょう。

Check the MedlinePlus Herbs and Supplements website yourself. It has information on many familiar items such as bilberry and blueberry, black and green tea, as well as calcium, magnesium and various vitamins.

☕ Relaxing a bit

次の英単語を、対応する日本語の単語に結びつけてみましょう。

1	Asian ginseng	・ ・	A	ザクロ
2	dandelion	・ ・	B	ウコン
3	eucalyptus	・ ・	C	ユーカリ
4	feverfew	・ ・	D	甘草
5	ginger	・ ・	E	朝鮮人参
6	licorice	・ ・	F	ナツシロギク
7	pomegranate	・ ・	G	生姜
8	turmeric	・ ・	H	タンポポ

Unit 4

Examining the source

　薬局で処方箋なしに購入できる市販薬を、英語でOver the Counter Medicine (OTC)といい、日本でも最近ではOTC薬とよんでいます。どんな薬がOTC薬になっているかは国によって違います。また、店内で客が自由に手に取って購入できるもの(off the shelf)と、カウンターの向こう側にいる薬剤師と話をしなければ手にできない、本当の意味でのOver the Counter Medicineとして制限のあるものなどもあり、OTC薬のあり方にも国により違いがあります。ここでは、OTC薬の箱を見てみましょう。

Getting to know the genre

図の中の文章を詳しく読む前に、次の1〜5に答えましょう。
Take a look at the text in the picture and answer the following questions.

1. What do you think this text is?

2. What is the purpose of the text?

3. Who is the audience for this text?

4. What kind of information does it give?

5. What are the language features of this text?

Reading the text → CD Track 06

front panel

side panel

PARACETAMOL+CODEINE+CAFFEINE COMBINATION

White chocolate flavour

PARACETAMOL+CODEINE+CAFFEINE COMBINATION

Fast acting, Powerful pain relief

Triple action analgesic
Paracetamol 500 mg, Codeine 8 mg, Caffeine 30 mg

Soluble powder, white chocolate flavour
24 sachets

Can cause addiction. For 3 days use only.

PARACETAMOL+CODEINE+CAFFEINE COMBINATION
Do not store above 30°C. Store in the original package.
Kodan Pharmaceutical Products Limited

back panel

PARACETAMOL+CODEINE+CAFFEINE COMBINATION
White chocolate flavour

PARACETAMOL+CODEINE+CAFFEINE COMBINATION
Do not store above 30°C. Store in the original package.
Kodan Pharmaceutical Products Limited

PARACETAMOL+CODEINE+CAFFEINE COMBINATION

For short term treatment of acute moderate pain when other painkillers have not worked.

For relief from:
migraine, tension headache, dental pain, menstrual period pain, backache and rheumatic pain.

Directions

How to take: For oral use. Pour one or two sachets of powder into a mug and fill with hot water (not boiling) and stir until dissolved. Milk can be added for milder taste.

How much to take: Adults and children 12 and over: 1 - 2 sachets every 4 hours. Do not take more than 8 sachets in any 24-hour period. Do not take for more than 3 days.

Ingredients

Ingredients (per sachet)	Action
Paracetamol 500 mg	Analgesic
Codeine phosphate 8 mg	Analgesic
Caffeine 30 mg	Enhances the analgesic effect

Also contains aspartame, sucrose and sodium. See leaflet for full list. Do not take if you have phenylketonuria.
This medicine may be harmful if you are on a low-sodium diet.

Warnings

CONTAINS PARACETAMOL. Do not take with any other paracetamol-containing products. Immediate medical advice should be sought in the event of an overdose, even if you feel well.
Contains codeine which can cause addiction if you take it continuously.
Do not take excessive amounts of tea, coffee or any other caffeine-containing drinks.
Do not take if you are pregnant or breast feeding.
If your symptoms persist and if you need to take it for more than 3 days, see your doctor or pharmacist for advice.

Read the enclosed leaflet carefully before use.
KEEP ALL MEDICINES OUT OF THE REACH AND SIGHT OF CHILDREN

注：音声には別の医薬品名が使われています。

❶ Checking the terms

GLOSSARY

addiction	[薬物への]依存、中毒	pain relief	鎮痛、疼痛緩和
analgesic	鎮痛剤、鎮痛の	paracetamol	パラセタモール（アセトアミノフェンの別名） ※解熱・鎮痛薬の一種
aspartame	アスパルテーム ※人工甘味料	persist	続く、持続する
backache	背痛、腰痛	pharmacist	薬剤師
breast feeding	授乳	pregnant	妊娠した
codeine phosphate	コデインリン酸塩、リン酸コデイン	rheumatic	リウマチの
dissolve	溶かす、溶解させる	sachet	[薬品などを包装した]小袋
enclosed	箱の中に入っている	sodium	ナトリウム
enhance	高める、強める	soluble	可溶性の、溶けやすい
excessive	過度の、必要以上の	sought	seek（[助言や解決策を]求める）の過去・過去分詞形
*flavour/flavor	味、風味、フレーバー	stir	[液体を]かき回す（混ぜる）こと
immediate	即刻の	sucrose	スクロース、ショ糖、白糖
leaflet	説明書	symptom	症状
**menstrual period pain	月経痛、生理痛	tension headache	緊張性（型）頭痛　※肩や首の筋肉の凝りからくる頭痛
migraine	片頭痛	treatment	治療、手当、医療
moderate pain	中程度の痛み	triple	3つの
overdose	[薬剤・麻薬の]過量（過剰）摂取		

*flavourはイギリス英語、flavorはアメリカ英語の綴りです。
**menstrual period painはmenstrual painやperiod painなど、省略して使われることもあります。

Learning the vocabulary

英語には痛み（疼痛）を表す語としてpain, ache, soreなどがあります。"Pain"は、けがや病気が原因で体に起きる痛みを表します。"Ache"は持続した不快で鈍い痛みを意味します。"Sore"はけがや感染または特定部位の酷使が原因で起こる痛みです。次の体の部分とpain, ache, soreのいずれかを組み合わせて痛みを適切に表現してみましょう。よく使われている組み合わせは1種類でないこともあります。辞書やインターネットで調べてみましょう

In English, there are many ways to describe "pain", for example, pain, ache and sore. "Pain" refers to physical suffering resulting from injury or illness. "Ache" is a pain which is not very strong but lasts a long time. "Sore" means pain or discomfort due to injury, infection or overuse of a muscle or part of the body. Complete the table below by combining a body part and "-pain", "-ache" and/or "sore-". Combinations may be more than one for each body part. Check dictionaries or websites to find the words combinations.

head	頭痛	headache
eyes【複】	目の痛み	①
ear	耳の痛み	②
tooth	歯痛	③
throat	喉の痛み	④
neck	首の痛み	⑤
shoulder	肩の痛み	⑥
chest	胸痛	⑦
stomach	胃痛, 腹痛	⑧
back	腰痛	⑨
muscle	筋肉痛	⑩
leg	足の痛み	⑪
knee	膝の痛み	⑫

Understanding the material

A) Paracetamol + Codeine + Caffeine Combinationの箱の表側を見てください。

Look at the front panel of the package of Paracetamol + Codeine + Caffeine Combination.

1) どんな薬ですか？

What kind of medicine is this?

2) 主成分は何ですか？

What are the main ingredients of this medicine?

3) 剤型は何でしょうか？どんな味がついていますか？

What is the form of this medicine? What is the flavour of this medicine?

4) 一箱に何包入っていますか？

How many sachets are in one box?

5) 重要な注意事項は何ですか？

What kind of warning is given?

B) 正面から見て箱の右の面にはどんな情報が書かれていますか？

What kind of information is written on the right panel of the box?

C) Paracetamol + Codeine + Caffeine Combinationの箱の裏側のラベルを見てください。この薬の説明は大きく分けて4つの項目 Directions, Ingredients, For relief from, Warningsからなっています。この薬を服用する際に知りたい情報（日本語）がこの4つのどれにあたるか、線で結びましょう。

Look at the label on the back panel of the Paracetamol + Codeine + Caffeine Combination package. The main information about this medicine consists of four parts: Directions, Ingredients, For Relief From, and Warnings. Which Japanese word below corresponds to the important information you need to know? Draw a line from the Japanese word to the English word.

1 成分・分量	·	·	A Warnings
2 用法・用量	·	·	B For relief from
3 効能・効果	·	·	C Ingredients
4 使用上の注意	·	·	D Directions

D) Paracetamol + Codeine + Caffeine Combinationの箱のラベル（表、裏、横）を見て1〜8の質問に対する答えを探し、(1)〜(14)をうめましょう。

Find the information to answer questions 1 - 8 from the Paracetamol + Codeine + Caffeine Combination package and fill in the blanks (1) – (14).

1. What kind of pain and symptoms can be relieved by Paracetamol + Codeine + Caffeine Combination?

   It can relieve (1)_____

   _____

   _____.

2. What is the maximum dosage of paracetamol in one day?

   The maximum dose is (2)_____ a day as the user can take up to (3)_____ a day and (4)_____ contains (5)_____ of paracetamol.

3. Which ingredient(s) may cause a severe effect if too much is taken at one time?

   It is (6)_____.

4. Why should Paracetamol + Codeine + Caffeine Combination not be taken for more than 3 days?

   It is because (7)_____ may cause an (8)_____.

5. What is the role of caffeine?

   The role of caffeine is to (9)_____ of (10)_____.

6. What is the form of this medicine and how do you take it?

   The form is (11)_____ and it is to be (12)_____ and taken as a (13)_____.

7. What are other ways of saying "painkiller"?

   They are (14)_____ and pain reliever.

8. What is the advice for the storage of Paracetamol + Codeine + Caffeine Combination?

   Paracetamol + Codeine + Caffeine Combination should be stored in (15)_____ and the storage temperature should not exceed (16)_____.

Note
薬の箱のラベルの内容や書き方は英語圏の国の間でも薬事法の違いにより書式や表現に違いがあることがあります。Paracetamol + Codeine + Caffeine Combinationはイギリスの一般的なOTC薬の表示の仕方に則っています。

Trying out the genre

ジェネリック医薬品 (generic medicine) という言葉を聞いたことはありますか？　ある薬の特許が切れると、同じ成分の薬が他社から安価で販売されるようになります。こういう薬がgeneric medicineとよばれるのです。日本語では後発医薬品ともよばれるため、genericとは「後発の」と

いう意味だと思われがちですが、このgenericという形容詞は、もともとは「一般的な」という意味です。薬にはbrand name/proprietary name（商品名/登録商標名）とその薬効成分を表すgeneric name/non-proprietary name（一般名）があります。ジェネリック医薬品（generic medicine）はしばしば商品名（brand name）ではなく一般名（generic name）で販売されます。文脈によってgenericの意味が異なることに注意しながら次の英文を読んでみましょう。英文はイギリス最大の健康情報を発信しているウェブサイトNHS Choicesからの抜粋です。

Why do medications have brand names and generic names?

Many medications have two names because more than one version of the medicine may be available.

- The brand name is the name given to a medicine by the pharmaceutical company that makes it. This is also called the proprietary name.
- The generic name or scientific name is the name for the active ingredient in the medicine that is decided by an expert committee and is understood internationally. This is also called the non-proprietary name.

Brand names for medications

Pharmaceutical companies take out a patent (exclusive rights) for each new medicine they discover. This patent lasts for up to 20 years, during which time the medicine is studied in clinical trials and then approved for sale by expert committees, such as the Medicines and Healthcare products Regulatory Agency (MHRA). When the medicine becomes available, only the pharmaceutical company that discovered it is able to sell it using their brand name, until the patent runs out.

Note
MHRAは、イギリス国内で販売・使用される医薬品と医療機器の安全性を管理するイギリスの政府機関です。

Generic names for medications

After the patent runs out, other companies can produce their own version of the medicine. For example, ibuprofen is the generic name of a medicine used to treat pain. Some companies will sell ibuprofen as branded versions, such as Nurofen and Hedex. Other manufacturers, such as Boots or Tesco, sell it under the generic name 'ibuprofen'.

Medicines sold under their generic name are usually cheaper because the research and development costs are lower. However, they contain the same active ingredient as the equivalent branded medicines.

NHS Choices
29/11/2012 より

上の文章を参考に Paracetamol + Codeine + Caffeine Combination の場合を考えてみましょう。下のa〜gから適切な語を選んで文章中の(1)〜(10)をうめましょう。brandとgenericは何度も使えます。

Now, think about the case of Paracetamol + Codeine + Caffeine Combination. Fill in the blanks with the appropriate word from the list below. The words "brand" and "generic" can be used as many times as necessary.

- a. brand
- b. consists of
- c. expired
- d. generic
- e. ingredients
- f. over-the-counter
- g. well-used

- Paracetamol + Codeine + Caffeine Combination is a medicine combination which (1)_____ three active well-known and (2)_____ ingredients. The (3)_____/non-proprietary names of these ingredients are paracetamol, codeine phosphate, and caffeine.

- Many companies make and sell this medicine combination because the patents of these three ingredients have (4) _____. Therefore, this is a (5) _____ medicine.
- This medicine is sold as an (6) _____ medicine (OTC) in many countries but is not available in Japan.
- Paracetamol is a (7) _____ name but it also has another (8) _____ name, acetaminophen, which is mainly used in North America (i.e. USA and Canada) and Japan.

Applying what you learned

Paracetamol + Codeine + Caffeine CombinationはイギリスのOTC薬の一般的なラベルでしたが、アメリカのラベルはどうなっているでしょうか？ アメリカのOTC薬のラベルは法律で書式が細かく決まっています。ここではアメリカのOTC薬のラベルの一例を"Throat Easy"という薬（トローチ）の箱を使ってみてみましょう。図を見て、1～9の空欄に当てはまる単語やフレーズを下のa～iから選び、正しい形にしてラベルを完成させましょう。

The Paracetamol + Codeine + Caffeine Combination package is written in the general UK style. Are there any differences between UK and US styles in the labeling? In the US, the OTC labeling format is strictly controlled by law. Let us examine an example of a US style label using the package of "Throat Easy" lozenges. Fill in the blanks 1-9 with appropriate words or phrases from the list below and complete the label.

a. allow lozenges to dissolve slowly in the mouth
b. ask a doctor
c. cherry flavor
d. do not use
e. glucose syrup
f. higher than 100°F
g. if pregnant or breast-feeding
h. protect from
i. oral anesthetic

> **Note**
> Throat Easyは架空の商品名です。

THROAT EASY
Cherry flavor 18 Lozenges

Soothing effective relief for sore throat

THROAT EASY
Cherry Flavor Lozenges

Benzocaine 10 mg, Cetylpyridinium chloride 2 mg

Oral Anesthetic, Analgesic and Antiseptic Action

18 Lozenges

Kodan Pharmaceutical Products Limited

Cherry flavor 18 Lozenges
THROAT EASY

Drug Facts

Active ingredients (per lozenge) | **Purpose**
Benzocaine 10 mg .... 1_____/Analgesic
Cetylpyridinium chloride 2 mg .... Antiseptic

Uses temporary relief of occasional
● sore throat, ● sore mouth   ● pain associated with canker sores
● minor mouth irritation

Warnings
2_____ if you have a history of allergy to local anesthetics such as procaine, butacaine, benzocaine or other "caine" anesthetics.
Stop use and 3_____ **if**
● sore throat is severe or lasts more than 2 days
● sore throat is accompanied or followed by fever, headache, rash, nausea or vomitting.
● sore mouth symptoms do not improve in 7 days
● irritation, pain or redness persists or worsens
Do not exceed recommended dosage.
4_____, ask a health professional before use.
Keep out of reach of children. In case of overdose, get medical help or contact a Poison Control Center right away.

Directions
● Adults and children 6 years of age and over. Take 1 lozenge every 2 hours as needed.
● 5_____
● Children under 6 years of age: Consult a doctor or dentist.

Other information
● Avoid storing at high temperature (6_____)
● 7_____ moisture.

Inactive ingredients Ascorbic acid, Carmoisine, 8_____,
Citric acid, 9_____, Sucrose, Tartaric acid, Zinc gluconate

Questions? 0-123-456-7890

Kodan Pharmaceutical Products Limited
THROAT EASY

---

1 (　　　)

2 (　　　)

3 (　　　)

4 (　　　)

5 (　　　)

6 (　　　)

7 (　　　)

8 (　　　)

9 (　　　)

Relaxing a bit

みなさんは今まで日本語で化学を学んできていますが、日本語で学んだ化学の用語は英語からの翻訳であったり、ドイツ語の発音をそのままカタカナにしたものがほとんどです。ここでは、基礎的な化学の用語を英語で見てみましょう。→ **CD Track 07**

1）よく使われる元素の名前

元素記号	element	元素	元素記号	element	元素
H	Hydrogen	水素	S	Sulfur	硫黄
C	Carbon	炭素	Cl	Chlorine	塩素
N	Nitrogen	窒素	K	Potassium	カリウム
O	Oxygen	酸素	Fe	Iron	鉄
Na	Sodium	ナトリウム	Cu	Copper	銅
P	Phosphorus	リン	Zn	Zinc	亜鉛

2）無機化合物の名前について

　無機・有機化合物の化学名はIUPAC (International Union of Pure and Applied Chemistry) 命名法に従って英語で命名します（日本薬局方準拠）。みなさんがよく知っている試薬の日本語名はそれらの訳ということになります。無機化合物のIUPAC名がどのように日本語に訳されているか例を見てみましょう。

　無機化合物の名前は、そこに含まれる元素イオンの名前を組み合わせて、命名されています。たとえばhydroxideというのは水酸化という意味ですが、

hydr-ox-ide → hydrogen(水素) + oxygen(酸素) + -ide(〜化) というようにです。

語尾	対応する日本語	例	IUPAC name 日本語名	化学式 chemical formula
-ide	〜化〜		Sodium hydroxide 水酸化ナトリウム	NaOH
-ate	〜酸〜塩		Calcium carbonate 炭酸カルシウム	$CaCO_3$
			Sodium hydrogen carbonate 炭酸水素ナトリウム	$NaHCO_3$
-ite	亜〜酸〜塩		Potassium nitrite 亜硝酸カリウム	KNO_2
-ic acid	〜酸		Sulfuric acid 硫酸	H_2SO_4
-ous acid	亜〜酸		Phosphorous acid 亜リン酸	H_3PO_3

IUPAC命名法については無機化学・有機化学の講義で詳しく触れると思いますので、よく勉強してください。

Unit 5

Examining the source

　英字新聞The Daily Yomiuriは、読売新聞社が提供する日刊英字紙で、国内で最大の発行部数を得ています。国内、国際、経済、ビジネス、スポーツ、科学、英語学習などの記事が掲載されています。また、提携紙としてワシントン・ポスト、ロサンゼルス・タイムズ、ザ・タイムズからの記事も読むことができます。オンライン版http://www.yomiuri.co.jp/dy/は、無料で利用可能です。新聞には、健康や医療に関する記事やコラムがしばしば掲載されています。

Getting to know the genre

テキストを詳しく読む前に次の1〜5に答えましょう。
Take a look at the text and find the answers to the following questions.

1. What do you think this text is?

2. What is the purpose of this text?

3. Who is the audience for this text?

4. What kind of information does it give?

5. What are the language features of this text?

Reading the text → CD Track 08

To Your Health / A spoonful of sugar makes the medicine go down

Maria was worried about her 3-year-old daughter Maya's 38°C temperature. She took her to the local clinic and left there with a shopping bag full of medicine, none of which she knew how to get Maya to take.

Maria had tablets, capsules and mysterious powders in tiny bags. Her first mistake was not insisting on knowing what each was for. Ordinarily, Japanese physicians will not explain medication unless asked, and if asked, they may be resentful of the implied distrust of their judgment. Ask anyway.

On the other hand, if a prescription is filled at a pharmacy, the pharmacist is usually more than happy to explain expected effects and possible side effects of the medicines, as well as offer advice about drug interactions and diet.

Foreigners are often surprised at the frequency with which powdered drugs are given in Japan. Japanese generally toss the dry powder into the back of their throats, and perhaps wash it down with water or tea. Foreigners tend to gag.

Diluting a powder in a liquid such as orange juice or dispersing it in a more palatable form such as strawberry jam makes it much easier to take. However, it is imperative to know if there are possible incompatibilities between drugs and foods. For example, the antibiotic tetracycline binds with the calcium in milk and is rendered useless.

Capsules are usually not prescribed for small children because of the obvious size reasons. Adults who have difficulty swallowing capsules should inform their doctor, as an alternative version may be available. Never open a capsule and attempt to down the contents. Capsules are designed to dissolve gradually, and taking the entire amount at one time could be hazardous.

Pills and tablets should also be treated with caution. Like capsules, some are coated to dissolve gradually in the digestive system. Breaking or crushing them to mix with something more palatable could be harmful. If you look at one and it is "scored," that is, has a mark down the middle, then it is safe to break it along this line.

It can't be said too many times—know what medicine you are taking (or giving your child) and if there are any special precautions.

If you are sure it is safe, and your child refuses or can't swallow solid medication, you can do what many Americans do and crush pills or tablets and mix the resulting powder with applesauce, jam, or flavored yogurt.

Knowing whether to take medication on an empty stomach or with food is also problematic. Instructions should be written on the label. This seemingly simple question can cause no end of confusion. For example, acetaminophen (Tylenol, paracetamol) works fastest on an empty stomach, but may be taken with food if it causes an upset stomach. Nonsteroid anti-inflammatory drugs (NSAIDs; aspirin, ibuprofen, naproxen, etc.) should generally be taken with food as they frequently cause indigestion.

Another consideration is adding a vitamin supplement to a pharmaceutical regimen that has kept one in balance for some time. An example that comes to mind is a woman who began taking a vitamin with iron after having been on a thyroid replacement for years, who found that her thyroid hormone level precipitously dropped.

Because drugs can so often interact with each other as well as food, be sure that each doctor you visit knows all the medications you are taking, including herbal remedies, and that you know how to administer drugs for optimal effect.

Note
paracetamolはacetaminophenの別名(一般名)です。Tylenolはacetaminophenを含む商品名で、多くの国でよく使われています。

Note
テキストは原文を尊重していますが、厳密にはNon-steroidal anti-inflammatory drugs (NSAIDs)と表記します。

THE DAILY YOMIURI, 2004年3月30日

Checking the terms

GLOSSARY

acetaminophen	アセトアミノフェン（パラセタモールの別名）※解熱・鎮痛薬の一種	interact	相互に作用する 【名】interaction　相互作用
administer	[薬などを]投与する	medication	薬剤、医薬品
alternative	別の可能性、代替手段(案)	naproxen	ナプロキセン ※解熱・鎮痛・抗炎症薬の一種
antibiotic	抗生物質		
aspirin	アスピリン ※解熱・鎮痛・抗炎症薬の一種	Non-steroidal anti-inflammatory drugs (NSAIDs)	非ステロイド性抗炎症薬 ※テキストは原文ママ
available	入手できる、利用できる	palatable	口当たりがいい
be rendered	～の状態にさせられる	paracetamol	パラセタモール（アセトアミノフェンの別名）※解熱・鎮痛薬の一種
bind with	結合する		
calcium	カルシウム	pharmacy	薬局
designed	設計された	physician	医師、医者、[総合]内科医
digestive system	消化器系	precaution	用心
dilute	[液体を]薄める、薄くする、希釈する	precipitously	急激に
		prescribe	処方する 【名】prescription　処方箋
disperse	分散させる、混ぜ込む		
dissolve	溶ける、溶解する	regimen	投薬計画
gag	息を詰まらせる	resentful	ひどく嫌がる
hazardous	有害な	supplement	栄養補助食品
ibuprofen	イブプロフェン ※解熱・鎮痛・抗炎症薬の一種	tablet	錠剤
		tetracycline	テトラサイクリン ※抗生物質の一種
incompatibility	不適合		
indigestion	消化不良	thyroid	甲状腺
instruction	使用説明書		

Learning the vocabulary

次のリストの単語およびフレーズから最も適当なものを選び、必要なら形を変えて、1から10までのセンテンスを完成させましょう。

Complete the following sentences with the best choice from the following list of terms.

antibiotic	empty stomach	side effects
available	indigestion	swallow
clinic	physician	
dissolve	prescription	

1. You can take this medicine on a full or (1)_____.
2. This medicine is commercially (2)_____ in Japan.
3. This vitamin pill takes about 30 to 45 minutes to (3)_____ in the stomach.
4. (4)_____ can occur if you eat too much.
5. In general, (5)_____ are small health facilities offering limited health services and short-term medical care.
6. The term (6)_____ often refers to a specialist in internal medicine and the term surgeon to a specialist in surgery.
7. (7)_____ are drugs that kill bacteria or slow their growth.
8. It is not easy to get children to (8)_____ pills and tablets.
9. Alcohol can trigger negative (9)_____ with some medicines.
10. The pharmacist will fill the (10)_____ for you right away.

Understanding the material

以下の1〜7を読んで、テキストの内容に当てはまるものにはT (true) を、当てはまらないものにはF (false)を、言及されていないものにはNS (not stated)を選びましょう。

Decide whether the following sentences are true (T), false (F), or not stated (NS) in the text.

1. Maria did not ask the doctor about the medication for Maya, but she knew what to do.   (   )
2. Powdered drugs are common outside of Japan.   (   )
3. Some tablets can be broken into small pieces to make them easier to take.   (   )
4. Many American parents give medicine to their children in ice cream.   (   )
5. Most medicines should be taken with food.   (   )
6. Supplements do not interact with drugs.   (   )
7. There are possible incompatibilities between drugs.   (   )

Trying out the genre

CDでインフルエンザに関する新聞記事の一部を聞いて、以下の空欄に適切な語を書き入れましょう。

→ CD Track 09

Listen to the reading of the following sentences in English from a news article about influenza. Write in the missing word in each blank.

　今期のインフルエンザワクチンは、A香港型とB型、3年前に発生した「インフルエンザ（H1N1）2009」の3種類が含まれる混合ワクチンで、現在の流行に対応している。

　だが、ワクチンは (1)_____ や気管支の免疫力を高めることはできても、主な感染経路となる (2)_____ や鼻などの粘膜には作用しないとされる。

　北里生命科学研究所の中山哲夫所長は「ワクチンは (3)_____ などの重症化を抑える作用はあるが、(4)_____ を防ぐのは難しい。過信せず、外出後の手洗いなどの (5)_____ を心がけてほしい」と話す。

　手洗いは、せっけんと流水で (6)_____ 秒以上かけて洗う。市販の速乾性 (7)_____ （濃度60〜80%）も、ウイルスを死滅させる力がある。

読売新聞2012年2月4日

📋 Applying what you learned

以下のようなシチュエーションで会話をつくって、ロールプレイしてみましょう。
Make a dialogue based on the following situation, and perform it as a role play.

薬剤師とお母さんの会話：
お母さんが子どもに、セフカプキシル（架空の抗生物質名）を服用させようとしますが、子どもがいやがります。薬剤師が次の2点の注意事項を含めたアドバイスをしています。
1. アイスクリームかヨーグルトに混ぜるといいが、オレンジ・パインジュースに混ぜると苦くなる。
2. 薬は散剤ではなく細粒剤であり、つぶすと苦くなる。

Roles: pharmacist and mother
The mother has to make her child take an antibiotic called Cefcapxil. The child does not like taking medicine. The pharmacist should tell the mother the following:
1. You can mix Cefcapxil with ice cream or yogurt, but not orange or pineapple juice because they make the medicine taste bitter.
2. This medicine is not a powder but is made of fine granules that should not be crushed.

☕ Relaxing a bit

　　国や地域によって、病気にかかったときなどの人々の対応はさまざまです。
高熱がでる⇒日本：布団掛けて、体を温め、汗をかいて、熱を下げる。
　　　　　　アメリカ：氷の入った水風呂に入る。
お腹が冷える（日本）⇒欧米の人には、「体を冷やすと病気になりやすい」というような
　　　　　　　　　概念がありません。
母乳の量を増やす方法⇒日本：おもちを食べる
　　　　　　　　アメリカ：ビールを飲む
　どちらも現在は医療従事者からは勧められていません。現代社会では食生活は豊かですから、おもちをたくさん食べると摂取カロリーが高くなりすぎます。ビールには実際、母乳を促進させると考えられる物質（a polysaccharide in the barley）が含まれていますが、アルコールは乳児には危険なものなので避けるべきです。

Unit 6

Examining the source

　このUnitでは、イギリスの高校生が使っている生物学の教科書を見てみましょう。イギリス（スコットランドを除く）の義務教育は5歳から17歳（2015年からは18歳）までです。大学に進学するためには17〜18歳の時に2年間かけて通称A-levelといわれる試験に向けて勉強し、AS level（1年目）とA2 level（2年目）を受験します。この結果は大学入学判定に使われ、薬学部に入学するためには、化学と生物学／数学／物理学の中から2科目（計3科目）を受験し、良い成績を取ることが条件になります。

Getting to know the genre

テキストを詳しく読む前に次の1〜5に答えましょう。
Take a look at the text and answer the following questions.

1. What do you think this text is?

2. What is the purpose of this text?

3. Who is the audience for this text?

4. What kind of information does it give?

5. What are the language features of this text?

Reading the text and understanding the material (1)

次の哺乳類の心臓に関するテキストを読み、図を見ながら空欄の(1)~(13)をうめましょう。
Read the following text and fill in the blanks 1-12 with the appropriate words from the diagram. → CD Track 10

The mammalian heart

The heart consists of a range of tissues. The most important one is cardiac muscle. The cells have the ability to contract and relax through the complete life of the person, without ever becoming fatigued. Each cardiac muscle cell is myogenic. This means it has its own inherent rhythm. Below are diagrams of the heart and its position in the circulatory system.

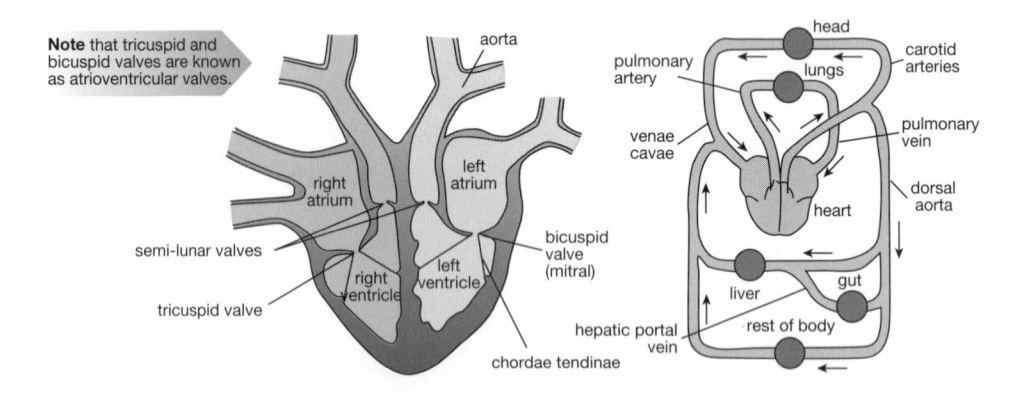

Structure

The heart consists of four chambers, right and left (1)_____ above right and left (2)_____ . The functions of each part are as follows.

- The right (3)_____ links to the right (4)_____ by the (5)_____ valve. This valve prevents backflow of the blood into the (6)_____ above,

when the (7) _____ contracts.
- The left (8) _____ links to the left (9) _____ by the (10) _____ valve (mitral valve). This also prevents backflow of the blood into the (11) _____ above.
- The chordae tendonae attach each (12) _____ to its (13) _____ valve.

Contractions of the ventricles have a tendency to force these valves up into the atria. Backflow of blood would be dangerous, so the chordae tendonae hold each valve firmly to prevent this from occurring.

- Semi-lunar (pocket) valves are found in the blood vessels leaving the heart (pulmonary artery and aorta). They only allow exit of blood from the heart through these vessels following ventricular contractions. Elastic recoil of these arteries and relaxation of the ventricles closes each semi-lunar valve.
- Ventricles have thicker muscular walls than atria. When each atrium contracts it only needs to propel the blood a short distance into each ventricle.
- The left ventricle has even thicker muscular walls than the right ventricle. The left ventricle needs a more powerful contraction to propel blood into the systemic circulation (all of the body apart from the lungs). The right ventricle propels blood to the nearby lungs. The contraction does not need to be so powerful.

If blood moved in the wrong direction, then transport of important substances would be impeded.

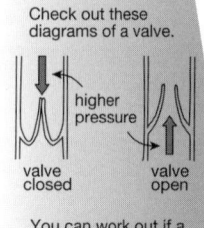

Check out these diagrams of a valve.

valve closed   valve open

higher pressure

You can work out if a valve is open or closed in terms of pressure. Higher pressure above than below a semi-lunar valve closes it. Higher pressure below the semi-lunar valve than above, opens it.

Revise AS and A2 Biology Complete Study and Revision Guide

Reprinted by permission of HarperCollins Publishers Ltd © 2008 John Parker and Ian Honeysett

Checking the terms

GLOSSARY

atrium	心房 【複】atria	inherent	本来備わっている、内在する
backflow	逆流	myogenic	筋原性の
cardiac muscle	心筋	occur	起こる、発生する
chordae tendinae / chordae tendonae	腱索（本UnitのRelaxing a bit 参照）	propel	進ませる
circulatory system	循環系	range	[同種で異なるものの] 集まり
consist of	～から成る、～で構成される	rhythm	リズム、律動
diagram	図表	valve	弁
exit	出ていくこと	ventricle	心室
fatigued	疲労した		

Learning the vocabulary

A) 英語には1つの単語に複数の意味を持つものがたくさんあります。下の表にまとめたrelaxation/relax, contraction/contract, allow（動詞のみ）はテキスト中で出てくる単語です。テキストでの意味とそのほかにどんな意味があるか（動詞形）、表の下のa)～h)から選んで表の(1)～(8)に入れましょう。それに対応する日本語を考えて表の(9)～(16)をうめましょう。

Many English words have more than one meaning. Look at the table below. Relaxation/relax, contraction/contract and allow (verb only) appear in the text. Think about the meanings of these words (in the verb form) in the text and in other situations, fill in the table by choosing the meanings from the list below.

名詞 Noun	動詞 Verb	Meanings		動詞の意味(日本語)
relaxation	relax	(1)		(9)
		(2)		(10)
contraction	contract	(3)		(11)
		(4)		(12)
contract		(5) e		(13)
	allow	(6)		(14)
		(7)		(15)
		(8)		(16)

a) to become ill

b) to rest while you are doing something enjoyable

c) to let somebody/something do something

d) to give permission

e) to make a legal agreement with someone to do work

f) to make something possible

g) to make or become shorter or narrower

h) to become or make something become less tight or stiff

B) 血液は心臓を出て血管を通って全身を巡り、心臓に戻ります。下の1～6は血管の名前です。対応する日本語とその血管を通る血液の流れる方向（図を見ながら）を線で結びましょう。

Blood leaves the heart, circulates the body through blood vessels and returns to the heart. Look at the names of the blood vessels 1-6 and match the most suitable Japanese name and direction of the blood flow by connecting the lines (hint: Check the diagrams).

Name of blood vessel		Japanese		direction of blood flow
1. pulmonary artery	·	· 肝門脈	·	· heart → lung
2. venae cavae	·	· 肺静脈	·	· gut → liver
3. hepatic portal vein	·	· 大静脈	·	· lung → heart
4. dorsal aorta	·	· 肺動脈	·	· heart → various regions
5. pulmonary vein	·	· 頸動脈	·	· heart → head, neck, brain
6. carotid artery	·	· 背部大動脈	·	· various regions → heart

Understanding the material (2)

次の1～4に答えましょう。

Answer the following questions.

Hint
See the note next to the main diagram

1. What do the chordae tendonae do in the heart?

2. Where are the semi-lunar valves located?

3. What types of valves are the atrioventricular valves?

4. Why is the muscle wall of the left ventricle thicker than that of the right ventricle?

Trying out the genre

次の文章は心臓発作に関する文章です。文章が意味をなすように、空欄(1)～(6)を次のa～fから選んだ言葉でうめましょう。

Read the following text about a heart attack. Fill in the each blank with the best word from the list to complete each sentence.

a. blood   c. muscle   e. symptoms
b. damage   d. myocardial infarction   f. the supply of blood

A heart attack is a serious medical emergency in which (1)_____ to the heart is suddenly blocked, usually by a blood clot. Lack of (2)_____ to the heart can seriously (3)_____ the heart (4)_____. A heart attack is known medically as a (5)_____ or MI.

(6) _____ can include:

- chest pain: the chest can feel like it is being pressed or squeezed by a heavy object, and pain can radiate from the chest to the jaw, neck, arms and back
- shortness of breath
- feeling weak and/or lightheaded
- overwhelming feeling of anxiety

It is important to stress that not everyone experiences severe chest pain; often the pain can be mild and mistaken for indigestion.

It is the combination of symptoms that is important in determining whether a person is having a heart attack, and not the severity of chest pain.

NHS Choices
13/03/2012より

Applying what you learned

脳卒中について調べ、空欄に入る語またはフレーズを a〜h から選んで文章を完成させましょう。
Complete the following text with the best choice from the list.

a. a blood vessel
b. may disappear
c. serious damage
d. serious medical emergency
e. speech
f. the face
g. to the brain
h. where the stroke occurs

A stroke is a (1)_____ in which the supply of blood (2)_____ is suddenly interrupted, usually due to a blood clot or the rupture of (3)_____. Lack of blood supply to an area of the brain can cause (4)_____.
The ability to speak, move or remember can be affected depending on (5)_____ in the brain.
Symptoms can include:
- drooping of one side of (6)_____
- the inability to raise an arm
- slurring of (7)_____

The symptoms (8)_____ in waiting for an ambulance to arrive but the person should be taken to the hospital for further checking.

Relaxing a bit

科学英語にはラテン語やギリシャ語由来の単語が多くあります。一般に英語では単数形を複数形にする時は、語尾に-sや-esをつけますが、ラテン語・ギリシャ語由来の英単語の場合は少し違います。このUnit 6に出てきた単語を含め、ラテン語・ギリシャ語由来の専門用語をいくつかご紹介します。

語尾変化	例(単数形)	例(複数形)	例(意味)
-um → -a	atrium	atria	心房
	medium	media	培地、媒体
	symposium	symposia	シンポジウム
	datum	*data	データ
-a → -ae	vena cava	venae cavae	大静脈
-on → -a	phenomenon	phenomena	現象
	mitochondrion	mitochondria	ミトコンドリア
-us → -i	hippocampus	hippocampi	海馬

*dataはdatumの複数形なので、本来その後に来る動詞は複数形に対応した形になるのですが、現在ではThis data is~という単数扱いで使うことが多く見られます。

Unit 6のテキスト中に出てきた腱索という単語は、chordae tendinaeを単数扱いchordae tendonaeを複数扱いにしてありますが、明確に使い分けられていないことがあります。またこの単語には別の綴りがあります。chorda tendinea【単】/chordae tendineae【複】です。ラテン語やギリシャ語由来の英単語にはそういった違う綴りのものがあります。ほかの例では髄芽腫という病気の英単語でmedulloblastomaとmedullablastomaという一字違いのものがあります。また、下の表にまとめているようにアメリカ式とイギリス式と認識されている綴りの違いもあります。

綴りの違い	単語例意味	アメリカ式	イギリス式
e ↔ ae	貧血	anemia	anaemia
	出血	hemorrhage	haemorrhage
	婦人科学	gynecology	gynaecology
	小児科学	pediatrics	paediatrics
e ↔ oe	下痢	diarrhea	diarrhoea
	胎児	fetus	foetus
	食道	esophagus	oesophagus
	エストロゲン	estrogen	oestrogen
o ↔ ou	腫瘍	tumor	tumour

Unit 7

Examining the source

　FDA (Food and Drug Administration of the United States Department of Health and Human Service) は、日本語で食品医薬品局といい、日本の厚生労働省にあたるアメリカ合衆国厚生省に属しています。アメリカ合衆国の「食品、薬品および化粧品に関する法律」の施行に携わる政府機関で、6つのセンターから成り立っています。そのうちの1つ、動物薬センター(Center for Veterinary Medicine (CVM)) は、動物用医薬品、動物由来食品、食品添加物の安全性・有効性を保証する機関です。このUnitのテキストは動物用医薬品センターからインターネット上で配信されている一般向けの健康に関する勧告です。

Getting to know the genre

本文を詳しく読む前に次の1～5に答えましょう。
Take a look at the text and answer the following questions.

1. What do you think this text is?

2. What is the purpose of this text?

3. Who is the audience for this text?

4. What kind of information does it give?

5. What are the language features of this text?

Reading the text → CD Track 11

Be Salmonella Safe!

1. What is *Salmonella*?
- *Salmonella* is a group of bacteria that can cause illness in people and animals.
- Salmonellosis is the name of the disease people and animals get from *salmonella* bacteria.
- *Salmonella* bacteria are tiny creatures that live in the intestines of animals (like turtles, snakes, lizards, frogs, salamanders, birds, and mice), and people.
- *Salmonella* can contaminate a variety of foods, such as meats, eggs, milk, seafood, vegetables, fruits, and even chocolate and peanut butter.
- The *Salmonella* bacteria can make people sick, especially young children, elderly people, and people with weak immune systems (like people with cancer).
- *Salmonella* was named after Daniel E. Salmon, a veterinarian who studied animal disease for the United States Department of Agriculture.

2. How do you get *Salmonella*?
- People can get Salmonella by eating foods contaminated by human or other animal poop. (For example, someone prepares a sandwich and does not wash his or her hands with soap and water after using the bathroom and then serves the sandwich to you. This can spread the Salmonella bacteria to you.)
- Eating raw or uncooked foods.
- Children can get Salmonella by kissing or holding

reptiles, baby birds, or other small animals.
- People can also get Salmonella after touching contaminated pet food or pet treats.

3. What are the symptoms of salmonellosis?
- In people, symptoms are diarrhea, fever, and stomach cramps. Symptoms can start 12-72 hours after infection and can last 4-7 days. Most people get better with only drinking more fluids.
- Some people (children, the elderly, and people with weak immune systems) are at high risk of bad infection and could die if they develop severe symptoms of Salmonella infection.
- Signs for pets include: vomiting, diarrhea (sometimes with blood), fever, not wanting to eat, not wanting to play, and laying around.

4. How can you be *Salmonella* Safe

You can be Salmonella Safe by remembering the following rules:
- Wash your hands with soap and water after touching animals (especially reptiles, birds, or amphibians), raw meat, poultry, or pet foods or treats.
- Cook poultry (like chicken or turkey), meat, hamburger, and eggs thoroughly.
- Don't eat or drink foods that have uncooked eggs or raw (unpasteurized) milk in them.
- If you are in a restaurant, send back all undercooked meat, poultry or eggs to the kitchen and have them cook it longer.
- Wash all kitchen work areas and utensils with soap and water right away after you have used them for cooking with raw meat or poultry.

- Wash your hands with soap and water after touching reptiles (like snakes or lizards), birds, amphibians (like frogs or salamanders), baby birds, or any pet poop.
- Keep reptiles (like turtles, iguanas, and snakes) away from babies, the elderly, or people with weak immune systems.
- Always wash your hands with soap and water before touching a baby (for example, to feed it or change its diaper), especially after you have touched any pets or uncooked poultry or meat.
- Wash your hands after going to the bathroom as well.

5. What is FDA doing to keep me *Salmonella* Safe?

   To Keep you Salmonella Safe, the Food and Drug Administration (FDA):

- inspects food production processes in the US
- inspects foods that come to the US from other countries
- makes sure that milk pasteurization plants are inspected
- makes sure that restaurants and factories that make different foods use good food handling techniques
- regulates how turtles are sold in the US, and
- regulates how certain antibiotics are used in food animals.

6. Who may I contact for more information?

- CVM (FDA Center for Veterinary Medicine):
  1-240-276-9300;1-888-INFO-FDA;AskCVM@fda.hhs.gov
- CFSAN (FDA Center for Food Safety and Nutrition):
  1-888-SAFEFOOD (1-888-723-3366)
- CDC (Centers for Disease Control):
  1-800-CDC-INFO (1-800-232-4636); cdcinfo@cdc.gov

FDA Center for Veterinary Medicineより

Checking the terms

GLOSSARY

amphibian	両生類	intestine	腸
antibiotic	抗生物質	lizard	トカゲ
bacteria	バクテリア、細菌【単】bacterium	poop	糞、便
contaminate	汚染する、不純にする	poultry	家禽、鳥肉、鶏肉
cramp	胃けいれん	regulate	規制する、制限する
creature	生き物、動物	reptile	は虫類
diarrhea	下痢	spread	広がる
feed	～に食物を与える	symptom	症状
fluid	液体	unpasteurized	低温殺菌処理されていない
immune systems	免疫機構	utensil	[主に台所の]器具、用具、用品
infection	感染	veterinarian	獣医
inspect	検査する、査察する	vomiting	嘔吐

Learning the vocabulary

次のリストの単語およびフレーズから最も適当なものを選び、必要なら形を変えて1～11のセンテンスを完成させましょう。

Here are some words and phrases that are useful to know. Choose the best word or phrase and change it to complete each sentence below.

antibiotic	diarrhea	regulate
at high risk for	inspect	symptom
contaminate	intestines	to make sure
develop	make you sick	

1. Healthcare professionals screen for patients (1) _____ diabetes in order to educate them about caring for themselves.
2. A runny nose can be a (2) _____ of a cold or allergy.
3. Dehydration was brought on by (3) _____.
4. The passage of food through the stomach and (4) _____ is illustrated in the textbook.
5. After the tanker accident, the oil that remained under the surface (5) _____ the water, plants and animals.
6. The city plans to (6) _____ the construction of high-rise buildings.
7. I checked several times (7) _____ the gas was turned off before I left the house.
8. If you eat food after the "use by" date, it may (8) _____.
9. The doctor gave the injured patient an (9) _____ to prevent infection.
10. While only a few (10) _____ the disease, it can cause brain damage or death.
11. (11) _____ the machine carefully before doing another experiment.

Understanding the material

次の1～8にセンテンスの形で答えましょう。

Answer the following questions with complete sentences.

1. What is *Salmonella*?

2. Name the hosts of *Salmonella* given in the text.

3. How does *Salmonella* enter the human body?

4. What symptoms are experienced if people are infected with *Salmonella*?

5. How long do the symptoms last?

6. Who are the most susceptible to *Salmonella*?

7. What should you do to protect against *Salmonella*?

8. What is FDA doing to keep people safe from *Salmonella*?

Trying out the genre

次の文はWikiopedia (http://en.wikipedia.org/wiki/Salmonellosis)からの抜粋で、2タイプのサルモネラ菌感染症、nontyphoidal form（非チフス型）とtyphoidal form（チフス型）について述べています。Typhoidal form（チフス型）の感染症について、この文をテキストのようなQuestion & Answerの形に変えてみましょう。

Here is an explanation of Salmonellosis from Wikipedia. It describes two types of Salmonella infection, a nontyphoidal form and a typhoidal form. Try rewriting the description of the typhoidal form as a Health Advisory, like that given above.

The type of Salmonella usually associated with infections in humans, **non typhoidal *Salmonella***, is usually contracted from sources such as:

- Poultry, pork, and beef, if the meat is prepared incorrectly or is infected with the bacteria after preparation.
- Infected eggs, egg products, and milk when not prepared, handled, or refrigerated properly.
- Reptiles, such as turtles, lizards, and snakes, which may carry the bacteria in their intestines.
- Tainted fruits and vegetables.

The typhoidal form of *Salmonella* can lead to typhoid fever. Typhoid fever is a life-threatening illness, and about 400 cases are reported each year in the United States, and 75% of these are acquired while traveling out of the country. It is carried only by humans and is usually contracted through direct contact with the fecal matter of an infected person. Typhoidal Salmonella is more commonly found in poorer countries, where unsanitary conditions are more likely to occur, and can affect as many as 21.5 million persons each year.

WIKIPEDIA, Salmonellosisより

📋 Applying what you learned

海外を旅行するにあたっては、必ずしも日本のように衛生状態のよい地域ばかりではありませんから、そうした場合には、準備にも注意が必要です。渡航前に感染症予防のためのワクチン接種が必要な場合もあります。旅行中、病気をしないために知っておくべきこともあります。CDC (http://wwwnc.cdc.gov/travel/) が有益な情報を提供しているので、旅行前にはチェックしてみましょう。検索は、地名でも病名でもできるようになっています。

If you plan to travel abroad, especially in areas where the hygiene conditions may not be as good as in Japan, you need to be particularly careful when preparing for your trip. Before you go, you may need vaccinations to prevent infection. While traveling, you need to know what precautions to take to stay healthy. One good place to check is the CDC (Centers for Disease Control and Prevention): http://wwwnc.cdc.gov/travel/ You can check the website according to your destination or by disease and find a lot of other useful information.

Relaxing a bit

日本語と英語での数字の増え方を比較して、英語での数字の読み方に慣れましょう。

日本語では、一、十、百、千の次は単位が万になり、万の前に一、十、百、千がつくことで数字が大きくなっていきます。次は単位が億に変わり、また、一、十、百、千を億の前につけますね。英語では、one, ten, hundredの次は単位がthousandになり、thousandの前にone, ten, hundredがついて、次は単位がmillionに変わります。millionの前にもone, ten, hundredをつけることで数字が大きくなってきます。hundred million（100,000,000）の次は単位がbillionに変わり、one, ten, hundred…とルール通りに増えていきます。

1	one	一
10	ten	十
100	hundred	百
1,000	one thousand	千
10,000	ten thousand	一万
100,000	hundred thousand	十万
1,000,000	one million	百万
10,000,000	ten million	千万
100,000,000	hundred million	一億

hundred millionの次はルールに沿って単位が変わりbillionになります。つまり、1,000,000,000 = one billionなのですが、実はこれはアメリカ式。イギリス・ヨーロッパ式では、別のルールに変わります。hundred millionの次はthousand millionと表し、billionはmillionが2つ（bi-）という意味で1,000,000,000,000（=10^{12}）のこと、trillionはmillionが3つ（tri-）という意味で1,000,000,000,000,000,000（=10^{18}）のことを表します。科学の世界ではアメリカ式で表しますが、そもそも科学では大きな数はone billionと表すより1×10^9 = one times ten to the power of nine/one times ten to the ninth/one times ten to the ninth powerと表すことが多いです。

ただし、現在では科学の世界以外でも英語圏の国ではアメリカ式 1,000,000,000（=10^9）= one billion、1,000,000,000,000（=10^{12}）= one trillionを公式には採用しています。ヨーロッパやほかの国々ではヨーロッパ式を採用したり、多言語が使用されている国では両方の方式が混在したりしています。

Unit 8

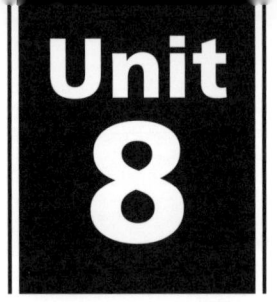

Examining the source

Centers for Disease Control and Prevention (CDC) アメリカ疾病管理予防センターはアメリカ合衆国保健福祉省管轄の感染症対策の機関です。感染症予防のための研究を行い、広くその情報を世界中に発信しています。

Getting to know the genre

テキストを詳しく読む前に次の1～5に答えましょう。
Take a look at the text and answer the following questions.

1. What do you think this text is?

2. What is the purpose of this text?

3. Who is the audience for this text?

4. What kind of information does it give?

5. What are the language features of this text?

Reading the text → CD Track 12

Hepatitis C Information for the Public

Overview

A: "Hepatitis" means inflammation of the liver. Toxins, certain drugs, some diseases, heavy alcohol use, and bacterial and viral infections can all cause hepatitis. Hepatitis is also the name of a family of viral infections that affect the liver; the most common types are Hepatitis A, Hepatitis B, and Hepatitis C.

B: Hepatitis A, Hepatitis B, and Hepatitis C are diseases caused by three different viruses. Although each can cause similar symptoms, they have different modes of transmission and can affect the liver differently. Hepatitis A appears only as an acute or newly occurring infection and does not become chronic. People with Hepatitis A usually improve without treatment. Hepatitis B and Hepatitis C can also begin as acute infections, but in some people, the virus remains in the body, resulting in chronic disease and long-term liver problems. There are vaccines to prevent Hepatitis A and B; however, there is not one for Hepatitis C. If a person has had one type of viral hepatitis in the past, it is still possible to get the other types.

C: Hepatitis C is a contagious liver disease that ranges in severity from a mild illness lasting a few weeks to a serious, lifelong illness that attacks the liver. It results from infection with the Hepatitis C virus (HCV), which is spread primarily through contact with the blood of an infected person. Hepatitis C can be either "acute" or "chronic."

Acute Hepatitis C virus infection is a short-term illness that occurs within the first 6 months after someone is exposed to the Hepatitis C virus. For most people, acute infection leads to chronic infection.

Chronic Hepatitis C virus infection is a long-term illness that occurs when the Hepatitis C virus remains in a person's body. Hepatitis C virus infection can last a lifetime and lead to serious liver problems, including cirrhosis (scarring of the liver) or liver cancer.

Transmission/Exposure

D: Hepatitis C is spread when blood from a person infected with the Hepatitis C virus enters the body of someone who is not infected. Today, most people become infected with the Hepatitis C virus by sharing needles or other equipment to inject drugs. Before 1992, when widespread screening of the blood supply began in the United States, Hepatitis C was also commonly spread through blood transfusions and organ transplants.

People can become infected with the Hepatitis C virus during such activities as

- Sharing needles, syringes, or other equipment to inject drugs
- Needlestick injuries in health care settings
- Being born to a mother who has Hepatitis C

Less commonly, a person can also get Hepatitis C virus infection through

- Sharing personal care items that may have come in contact with another person's blood, such as razors or toothbrushes
- Having sexual contact with a person infected with the Hepatitis C virus

Symptoms

E: Approximately 70–80% of people with acute Hepatitis C do not have any symptoms. Some people, however, can have mild to severe symptoms soon after being infected, including

- Fever
- Fatigue

- Loss of appetite
- Nausea
- Vomiting
- Abdominal pain
- Dark urine
- Clay-colored bowel movements
- Joint pain
- Jaundice (yellow color in the skin or eyes)

F: Most people with chronic Hepatitis C do not have any symptoms. However, if a person has been infected for many years, his or her liver may be damaged. In many cases, there are no symptoms of the disease until liver problems have developed. In persons without symptoms, Hepatitis C is often detected during routine blood tests to measure liver function and liver enzyme (protein produced by the liver) level.

G: Chronic Hepatitis C is a serious disease that can result in long-term health problems, including liver damage, liver failure, liver cancer, or even death. It is the leading cause of cirrhosis and liver cancer and the most common reason for liver transplantation in the United States. Approximately 15,000 people die every year from Hepatitis C related liver disease.

Treatment

H: There is no medication available to treat acute Hepatitis C infection. Doctors usually recommend rest, adequate nutrition, and fluids.

I: Each person should discuss treatment options with a doctor who specializes in treating hepatitis. This can include some internists, family practitioners, infectious disease doctors, or hepatologists (liver specialists). People with chronic Hepatitis C should be monitored regularly for signs of liver disease and evaluated for treatment. The treatment most often used for Hepatitis C is a combination of two medicines, interferon and ribavirin. However, not every person with chronic Hepatitis C needs or will benefit from treatment. In addition, the drugs may cause serious side effects in some patients.

Centers for Disease Control and Prevention (CDC), 01/17/2013より

Checking the terms

GLOSSARY

abdominal	腹部の	interferon	インターフェロン、ウイルス抑制因子
acute	急性の	internist	内科医
affect	~に害を及ぼす、~に影響を及ぼす	mode	方法
approximately	およそ、約、だいたい、~前後	nausea	吐き気、悪心
bowel	腸	nutrition	栄養
chronic	慢性の	primarily	第一に、主として
cirrhosis	肝硬変	ribavirin	リバビリン ※抗肝炎ウイルス薬の一種
contagious	伝播する、伝染する、伝播性の、伝染性の	scarring	瘢痕化
exposed to	~にさらされる、曝露する	symptom	症状
fatigue	疲れ、疲労、けん怠感	transmission	伝播、伝染、感染
hepatitis	肝炎	transplantation	移植
hepatologist	肝臓専門医	urine	尿
infection	感染、感染症	vaccine	ワクチン
inflammation	炎症	viral	ウイルス性の
inject	~を注射する	widespread	広がった、及んでいる、まん延した

Learning the vocabulary

A) テキスト中に出てきた下線を引いてある単語「inflammation（名詞）」「infection（名詞）」「transmission（名詞）」「expose（動詞）」を動詞形、名詞形、形容詞形に変化させて下の表を完成させましょう。答えが2つあるものもあります。

Look at the "Reading the text" section and find the underlined words. Change the form of the underlined words: *inflammation* (noun), *infection* (noun), *transmission* (noun), *expose* (verb) to verb, noun or adverb forms and fill in the table below. There may be more than word that fits in some of the boxes.

Verb (動詞)	Noun (名詞) 右の欄は日本語を入れましょう		Adjective (形容詞)
	inflammation		
	infection		
	transmission		
expose			exposed

B) 左側には病気の症状を説明するときに使う単語が、右側にはそれらのほかのいい方や説明文が書かれています。左側の単語に合う右側の説明文を線でつなぎましょう。

Words to describe symptoms are listed on the left hand side. On the right hand side are alternative words and/or an explanation of those words. Draw a line to connect a word on the left hand side with the appropriate word or explanation on the right hand side.

1 acute	**A**	stomachache
2 chronic	**B**	be sick, throw up, to bring food from the stomach back out through the mouth
3 fatigue	**C**	physical desire for food
4 nausea	**D**	quick, severe, short-time
5 vomit	**E**	persistent, long-term
6 abdominal pain	**F**	feeling sick, feeling when you want to vomit
7 appetite	**G**	a feeling of being extremely tired

Understanding the material

A) 下の1〜9はテキストのパラグラフA~Iの見出しです。1〜9の見出しはそれぞれA〜Iのうちいずれの見出しとして最適か選びましょう。

Which following titles 1 – 9 best fit paragraphs A – I?

1. What is the difference between Hepatitis A, Hepatitis B, and Hepatitis C?　　　　　　　　　　パラグラフ_____

2. What are the symptoms of chronic Hepatitis C?
　　　　　　　　　　　　　　　　　　　パラグラフ_____

3. How is acute Hepatitis C treated?　　パラグラフ_____

4. What are the symptoms of acute Hepatitis C?
　　　　　　　　　　　　　　　　　　　パラグラフ_____

5. How is chronic Hepatitis C treated?　パラグラフ_____

6. What is hepatitis?　　　　　　　　　パラグラフ_____

7. How serious is chronic Hepatitis C?　パラグラフ_____

8. How is Hepatitis C spread?　　　　　パラグラフ_____

9. What is Hepatitis C?　　　　　　　　パラグラフ_____

B) 以下の1～7を読んで、テキストの内容に当てはまるものにはT (true) を、当てはまらないものにはF (false)を、言及されていないものには NS (not stated)を選びましょう。Fの場合には、間違っている内容をセンテンスの形で書き直しましょう。

Decide whether the following sentences are true (T), false (F), or not stated (NS) in the text. If your answer is F, then rewrite the sentence as a true one.

1. Hepatitis is caused only by virus infection.　　　(　　)

2. Hepatitis A, B and C all develop from the acute to the chronic stage.　　　(　　)

3. Only hepatitis B can be prevented by a vaccine.　　　(　　)

4. A person can be infected by several types of hepatitis viruses.　　　(　　)

5. A child of a mother infected with hepatitis C is at a risk of getting hepatitis C infection.　　　(　　)

6. Many patients with chronic hepatitis C notice their illness from symptoms such as fever, fatigue, loss of appetite, and so on.　　　(　　)

7. Hepatitis D, caused by the hepatitis D virus, is only present in people already infected with hepatitis B.   (   )

Trying out the genre

次の文章はNHS (National Health Service) が提供するウェブサイト
http://www.nhs.uk/conditions/hepatitis-c/pages/treatment.aspx
からの抜粋で、C型肝炎の治療薬について述べています。説明の中の空欄(1)～(6)に当てはまる言葉を次のa～fから選び、書き入れましょう。

The following sentences are extracts from an NHS website giving information about the drugs used for hepatitis C treatment. Fill in the blanks with words from the table to complete the sentences.

Note
*pegylated: ペグ化した
ペグ化したインターフェロンとは、インターフェロンα (2aや2bなど製薬会社によって違うタイプがある) を高分子のポリエチレングリコール (PEG) で覆うことによって血中からの消失半減期を延長させたもの。従来のインターフェロン製剤が毎日～週3回投与であるのに対し、ペグ化インターフェロンは週1回の投与でよいので、患者の通院の負担は軽減される。

NHS Choices, 29/12/2011より

a. antiviral   c. occurring   e. stimulates
b. capsule or tablet d. spreading   f. synthetic

Treatment for chronic hepatitis C usually involves using a combination of two medication:
- *pegylated interferon (given as an injection) – a (1)____ version of a naturally (2)____ protein in the body that (3)____ the immune system to attack virus cells
- ribavirin (given as a (4)____) – a type of (5)____ drug that stops hepatitis C from (6)____ inside the body

This is known as combination therapy.

📋 Applying what you learned

次の文はテキストと同じくCDCのウェブページにあげられているもので、インフルエンザに関する情報です。読んだ後、質問1～5に答えましょう。

Here is the information from CDC webpage on Influenza. Apply what you have learned to understand the following passage. Answer the questions below.

Influenza Type A Viruses and Subtypes

There are three types of influenza viruses: A, B and C. Human influenza A and B viruses cause seasonal epidemics, generally between October and May, of disease in the United States.

Wild aquatic birds are the natural hosts for all known influenza type A viruses - particularly certain wild ducks, geese, swans, gulls, shorebirds and terns. Influenza type A viruses can infect people, birds, pigs, horses, dogs, marine mammals, and other animals. Influenza type A viruses are divided into subtypes on the basis of two proteins on the surface of the virus: hemagglutinin (HA) and neuraminidase (NA). For example, an "H7N2 virus" designates an influenza A virus subtype that has an HA 7 protein and an NA 2 protein. Similarly an "H5N1" virus has an HA 5 protein and an NA 1 protein. There are 17 known HA subtypes and 10 known NA subtypes. Many different combinations of HA and NA proteins are possible. All known subtypes of influenza A viruses can infect birds, except subtype H17N10 which has only been found in bats. Only two influenza A virus subtypes (i.e., H1N1, and H3N2) are currently in general circulation among people. Some subtypes are found in other infected animal species. For example, H7N7 and H3N8 virus infections can cause illness in horses, and H3N8 virus infection can also cause illness in dogs.

Avian influenza A viruses are classified into two categories (low pathogenic and highly pathogenic) that refer to their ability to cause severe disease, based upon molecular characteristics of the virus and mortality in birds under experimental conditions. Infection of poultry with low pathogenic avian influenza A (LPAI) viruses may cause no disease or mild illness (such as ruffled feathers and a drop in egg production) and may not be detected. Infection of poultry with highly pathogenic avian influenza A (HPAI) viruses can cause severe disease with high mortality. Both HPAI and LPAI viruses can spread rapidly through poultry flocks. HPAI virus infection can cause disease that affects multiple internal organs with mortality up to 90-100% in chickens, often within 48 hours. However, ducks can be infected without any signs of illness. There are genetic and antigenic differences between the influenza A virus subtypes that typically infect only birds and those that can infect birds and people.

Centers for Disease Control and Prevention (CDC), March 22, 2012 より

Questions on passage

1. How many types of influenza viruses are there?

2. What kind of animal is the natural host of influenza A viruses?

3. What other animals can influenza A viruses infect?

4. What does H5N1 mean?

5. What subtypes are known to infect humans?

Relaxing a bit

　Unit 8 では、肝炎ウイルスやインフルエンザウイルスについて触れました。ここでウイルスの発見についてのお話を。

　医学の研究は、顕微鏡が発明されたおかげで大きく発展しました。17世紀の半ばから顕微鏡を使って、病気の原因となる微生物が目に見えるようになり、コレラ・チフスなど恐ろしい急性伝染病と、結核・梅毒などの慢性伝染病の病原体が次々に発見されました。

　しかし19世紀末になって、顕微鏡で目に見えるこれら細菌以外にも、ヒトに感染して病気を起こす病原体があることが明らかになってきたのです。瀬戸物の土台となる、顔料をかけていない素焼きの器があります。植木鉢がその代表ですが、細かい隙間があって細菌を通さないために、飲料水の消毒のためにも使われていました。しかし、細菌を除いたはずのこの器で濾過した水を飲んだ後にも病気が起こることがわかったのです。これを「濾過性病原体」とよんでいましたが、のちに別名でラテン語の「毒」を表すウイルスといわれるようになりました。

　このように、ウイルスの最大の特徴は「小さいこと」と「感染性がある」という2点です。細菌の代表で、O-157変種のために数年前に大問題となった大腸菌は、直径1ミクロン弱で長さ3ミクロンほどの大きさがあります。1ミクロンは1ミリの千分の1の単位ですから、ずいぶん小さな生物で、顕微鏡で400倍に拡大してやっと見える程度の大きさです。一方、ウイルスは細菌と比べてずっと小さくその十分の1から百分の1くらいの大きさしかありません。20世紀半ばに電子顕微鏡が発明されて、ウイルスを1万倍も拡大することができるようになって、やっとあらゆるウイルスの本体を見ることができるようになりました。そういうわけで、ウイルスの大きさを測るには1ミクロンのさらに千分の1に相当する1ナノメーター（百万分の1ミリに相当します）という単位が使われています。

　ウイルスがどのくらい小さいかを実感するために、こんな比較がされています。人体に地球の大きさがあると仮定すると、ウイルスはせいぜい「象さん」くらいの大きさにしかならないのだそうです。地球の大きさと象の大きさを思い比べてみると、ウイルスがいかに小さいかが、よくわかりますよね。

（参照：http://www.tokumen.co.jp/column/kanzo1/02.html）

Unit 9

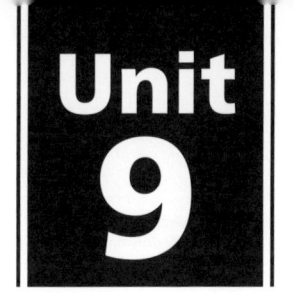

Examining the source

　食品医薬品局（FDA; Food and Drug Administration）は、消費者が通常の生活を行うにあたって接する機会のある製品について、その許可や違反品の取締りなどの行政を専門的に行うアメリカ合衆国の政府機関です。扱う品目は、食品や医薬品、さらに化粧品、医療機器、動物用医薬品、玩具など多岐にわたります。このUnitでは、FDAが提供する、化粧品・医薬品および石けんに関する法律上の情報を読みましょう。

Getting to know the genre

本文を詳しく読む前に次の1～5に答えましょう。
Take a look at the text and answer the following questions.

1. What do you think this text is?

2. What is the purpose of this text?

3. Who is the audience for this text?

4. What kind of information does it give?

5. What are the language features of this text?

Reading the text → CD Track 13

Is It a Cosmetic, a Drug, or Both? (Or Is It Soap?)

July 8, 2002; updated April 30, 2012

Whether a product is a cosmetic or a drug under the law is determined by a product's intended use. Different laws and regulations apply to each type of product. Firms sometimes violate the law by marketing a cosmetic with a drug claim or by marketing a drug as if it were a cosmetic, without adhering to requirements for drugs.

How does the law define a cosmetic?

The Federal Food, Drug, and Cosmetic Act (FD&C Act) defines cosmetics by their intended use, as "articles intended to be rubbed, poured, sprinkled, or sprayed on, introduced into, or otherwise applied to the human body...for cleansing, beautifying, promoting attractiveness, or altering the appearance" [FD&C Act, sec. 201(i)]. Among the products included in this definition are skin moisturizers, perfumes, lipsticks, fingernail polishes, eye and facial makeup preparations, cleansing shampoos, permanent waves, hair colors, and deodorants, as well as any substance intended for use as a component of a cosmetic product.

How does the law define a drug?

The FD&C Act defines drugs, in part, by their intended use, as "articles intended for use in the diagnosis, cure, mitigation, treatment, or prevention of disease" and "articles (other than food) intended to affect the structure or any function of the body of man or other animals" [FD&C Act, sec. 201(g)(1)].

How can a product be both a cosmetic and a drug?

Some products meet the definitions of both cosmetics and drugs. This may happen when a product has two intended uses. For example, a shampoo is a cosmetic because its intended use is to cleanse the hair. An antidandruff treatment is a drug because its intended use is to treat dandruff. Consequently, an antidandruff shampoo is both a cosmetic and a drug. Among other cosmetic/drug combinations are toothpastes that contain fluoride, deodorants that are also antiperspirants, and moisturizers and makeup marketed with sun-protection claims. Such products must comply with the requirements for both cosmetics and drugs.

How is a product's intended use established?
Intended use may be established in a number of ways. The following are some examples:
- Claims stated on the product labeling, in advertising, on the Internet, or in other promotional materials.

Certain claims may cause a product to be considered a drug, even if the product is marketed as if it were a cosmetic.

- **Consumer perception, which may be established through the product's reputation.** This means asking why the consumer is buying it and what the consumer expects it to do.
- **Ingredients that cause a product to be considered a drug because they have a well-known (to the public and industry) therapeutic use.** An example is fluoride in toothpaste.

How are the laws and regulations different for cosmetics and drugs?

How approval requirements are different

Under the FD&C Act, cosmetic products and ingredients, with the exception of color additives, do not require FDA approval before they go on the market. Drugs, however, must generally either receive premarket approval by FDA through the New Drug Application (NDA) process or conform to a "monograph" for a particular drug category, as established by FDA's Over-the-Counter (OTC) Drug Review. These monographs specify conditions whereby OTC drug ingredients are generally recognized as safe and effective, and not misbranded.

How good manufacturing practice requirements are different

Good manufacturing practice (GMP) is an important factor in helping to assure that your cosmetic products are neither adulterated nor misbranded. However, while FDA has provided guidelines for cosmetic GMP (see "Good Manufacturing Practice (GMP) Guidelines/ Inspection Checklist"), no regulations set forth specific GMP requirements for cosmetics. In contrast, the law requires strict adherence to GMP requirements for drugs, and there are regulations specifying minimum current GMP requirements for drugs [Title 21 of the Code of Federal Regulations (CFR), parts 210 and 211]. Failure to follow GMP requirements causes a drug to be adulterated [FD&C Act, sec. 501(a)(2)(B)].

How registration requirements are different
FDA maintains the Voluntary Cosmetic Registration Program, or VCRP, for cosmetic establishments and formulations [21 CFR 710 and 720]. As its name indicates, this program is voluntary. The FD&C Act does not require cosmetic firms to register their establishments or list their product formulations with FDA. In contrast, it is mandatory for drug firms to register their establishments and list their drug products with FDA [FD&C Act, sec. 510; 21 CFR 207]. See Drug Listing and Registration System (DRLS and eDRLS).

How labeling requirements are different
A cosmetic product must be labeled according to cosmetic labeling regulations. See the Cosmetic Labeling Manual for guidance on cosmetic labeling and links to the regulations related to cosmetic labeling. OTC drugs must be labeled according to OTC drug regulations, including the "Drug Facts" labeling, as

described in 21 CFR 201.66. Combination OTC drug/cosmetic products must have combination OTC drug/cosmetic labeling. For example, the drug ingredients must be listed alphabetically as "Active Ingredients," followed by cosmetic ingredients, listed in descending order of predominance as "Inactive Ingredients."

And what if it's "soap"?

Soap is a category that needs special explanation. That's because the regulatory definition of "soap" is different from the way in which people commonly use the word. Products that meet the definition of "soap" are exempt from the provisions of the FD&C Act because—even though Section 201(i)(1) of the act includes "articles... for cleansing" in the definition of a cosmetic—Section 201(i)(2) excludes soap from the definition of a cosmetic.

How FDA defines "soap"

Not every product marketed as soap meets FDA's definition of the term. FDA interprets the term "soap" to apply only when

- the bulk of the nonvolatile matter in the product consists of an alkali salt of fatty acids and the product's detergent properties are due to the alkali-fatty acid compounds, and
- the product is labeled, sold, and represented solely as soap [21 CFR 701.20].

Products that meet this definition of soap are regulated by the Consumer Product Safety Commission (CPSC), not by FDA. Please direct questions about these products, such as [safety and] labeling requirements, to CPSC.

U. S. Food and Drug Administration, April 30, 2012 より

Checking the terms

GLOSSARY

additive	添加物	dandruff	ふけ
adhere/adherence	順守する/順守	define	定義する
adulterate	品質を落とす、不良品の	diagnosis	診断、診断結果
affect	〜に作用する、〜に影響する	evaluation	評価
alter	変える	exclude	〜を除く、除外する、抜かす
antidandruff	ふけ予防の	fatty acid	脂肪酸
antiperspirant	制汗剤	function	機能
apply	適用する、塗る	guideline	指針
article	品物、商品	ingredient	原料、材料、成分
assure	〜を保証する	interpret	解釈する、説明する
claim	宣伝文句、主役	labeling	表示
comply	従う	mandatory	必須の、義務的な
component	構成要素	misbranded	不正商標表示の
compound	化合物	mitigation	緩和
conform	従う、守る	nonvolatile	不揮発性の
consist	[〜から]成る	perception	認知、見識、感じ方
consumer	消費者	predominance	数量的優勢
cure	治療法、治癒	regulation	規則、法規、法令
		requirement	要件

rub	こする	structure	構造
specify	～を明確に述べる	violate	[法律・契約などに]違反する
sprinkle	振りかける	voluntary	任意の

Learning the vocabulary

次のリストの単語から最も適当なものを選んで1から11までのセンテンスを完成させましょう。
Here are some words that are useful to know. Choose the best word or phrase to complete each sentence below.

adhere	apply	consist	interpret
affect	assure	define	specify
alter	conform	exclude	violate

1. How would you (1) _____ "happiness"?
2. I can (2) _____ you that all will go well.
3. How do you (3) _____ these sentences?
4. Drunkenness may (4) _____ a person's behavior.
5. There will be chaos unless we all (5) _____ to the rules.
6. After washing your face with the soap, rinse it off with water, and (6) _____ lotion to the skin.
7. The amount of rain will (7) _____ the growth of crops.
8. Would you like to (8) _____ any day or time-slot for your delivery?
9. You should (9) _____ to the customs of the country.
10. Those who (10) _____ the rules will be punished.

11. Taxes (11) _____ of direct taxes and indirect ones.
12. Mosquito nets should be made so that they (12) _____ insects but allow air to pass.

Understanding the material

次の各問いにセンテンスの形で答えましょう。

Answer the following questions with complete sentences.

1. What determines whether a product is a cosmetic or a drug under the law?

2. How does the FDA define cosmetics?

3. Name some of the products that are defined as cosmetics.

4. How does the FDA define drugs?

5. On what basis is an antidandruff defined (a) as a cosmetic and (b) as a drug?

6. Name three examples of ways that intended use is established.

7. Explain the process in which drugs can obtain FDA approval before going on the market.

8. How do cosmetics and drugs differ in terms of requirements regarding good manufacturing practice (GMP)?

9. How does the FDA define "soap"?

Trying out the genre

　このテキストの文書は一般の人々を対象としていますが、文書中に多く含まれている固有名詞を知らないままでは、理解するのが難しい箇所があります。次の固有名詞をインターネットで調べてみましょう。

This text is for a general public audience but has many proper nouns which can make it difficult to understand. Check websites or other resouces to find out what they mean.

- New Drug Application (NDA)

- Over-the-Counter (OTC) Drug Review

- Good Manufacturing Practice (GMP)

- Consumer Product Safety Commission (CPSC)

Applying what you learned

A) 次の文は、日本の厚生労働省医薬食品局が発行する文書（平成12年発行、平成23年一部改正）の英語版Regulation of Cosmetics in Japanからの抜粋で、化粧品を定義する文です。FDAのものと似ている点、異なる点を話しあってみましょう。

The following text is from the Regulation of Cosmetics in Japan. It gives the definition of a "cosmetic". Compare this text with the FDA text and discuss the similarities and differences.

Article 2-3 of the Pharmaceutical Affairs Act: Under this law, "cosmetic" refers to any item having mild effects on the human body that is rubbed, spread, or otherwise applied in a similar manner for the purpose of cleansing, beautifying, or enhancing the attractiveness of the human body, to change physical appearance, or to maintain skin or hair in a healthy condition. (Examples: Beauty lotion, perfume, soap, toothpaste, lipstick, shampoo, bath additive, hair manicure, etc.)

http://documents.eu-japan.eu/seminars/japan/ja/dataobj-374-datafile.pdfより

B) また、下にあげる同文書の「化粧品の効能の範囲」の日本語版の抜粋を読み、FDAの規定する化粧品の効能の範囲と似ている点、異なる点を話しあってみましょう

Compare the Japanese explanation of the effects of cosmetics with the FDA description.

①頭皮、毛髪を清浄にする。　②香りにより毛髪、頭皮の不快臭を抑える。　③頭皮、毛髪をすこやかに保つ。　④毛髪にはり、こしを与える。　⑤頭皮、毛髪にうるおいを与える。　⑥頭皮、毛髪のうるおいを保つ。　⑦毛髪をしなやかにする。　⑧クシどおりをよくする。　⑨毛髪のつやを保つ。　⑩毛髪につやを与える。　⑪フケ、カユミがとれる。　⑫フケ、カユミを抑える。　⑬毛髪の水分、油分を補い保つ。　⑭裂毛、切毛、枝毛を防ぐ。　⑮髪型を整え、保持する。　⑯毛髪の帯電を防止する。

Relaxing a bit

Unit 9のテキスト中に出てくる法令名は、どのように読むでしょうか。 → CD Track 14

FD&C Act, sec. 201(g)(1)

 Federal Food, Drug, and Cosmetic Actは長すぎるので以下のように読みます．

 F D and C Act section two zero one g one

 アルファベットをひとつずつ読み、& (ampersand) は"and"と読みます。"sec."は"section"です。あとはアルファベットと数字をひとつずつ読みます。

FD&C Act, sec. 510

 F D and C Act section five one zero (ほかの読み方として five one oh, five ten ; 0 を"oh"としてよく読みますが、音が"four"に近いので間違いのないように"zero"として読むことを勧めます)

FD&C Act, sec. 501(a)(2)(B)

 F D and C Act section five zero one a two capital B (小文字はそのまま、大文字は capital を前につけて読みます)

21 CFR 207

 Title 21 Code of Federal Regulations part two zero seven

 Title 21 C F R part two zero seven (two oh seven とも読みます)

21 CFR 201.66

 Title 21 Code of Federal Regulations part two zero one point six six (two oh one point six six)

 Title 21 C F R part two zero one point six six

Section 201(i)(2)

 Section two zero one i two (two oh one i two)

Unit 10

Examining the source

　The New England Journal of Medicine（略称：N Engl J Med または NEJM）は、マサチューセッツ内科外科学会が発行する査読制の医学雑誌です。医学系定期刊行物の中では世界で最も長い歴史を誇り、最も広く読まれ、また最もよく引用され、強い影響力を持っています。研究論文、臨床報告、総説など医療従事者を対象読者とする専門性の高い学術文書がおもな構成内容ですが、医療やそれに関連する社会問題についての幅広いトピックをカバーする記事も含み、それらの中には高度専門知識がなくとも充分に読みこなせるものもあります。この Unit で取りあげるのは、アメリカのロードアイランド州プロビデンスにある介護施設でセラピーキャットとして暮らす不思議な能力を持った猫の話です。著者ドーサ氏は、同施設の回診に来ていた老人医療の専門医です。

Getting to know the genre

テキストを詳しく読む前に次の 1 ～ 5 に答えましょう。
Take a look at the text and answer the following questions.

1. What is the genre of this text?

2. What is the purpose of this text?

3. Who is the audience for this text?

4. What kind of information does it give?

5. What are the language features of this text?

Reading the text → CD Track 15

A Day in the Life of Oscar the Cat

David M. Dosa, M. D., M.P.H.

Oscar the Cat awakens from his nap, opening a single eye to survey his kingdom. From atop the desk in the doctor's charting area, the cat peers down the two wings of the nursing home's advanced dementia unit. All quiet on the western and eastern fronts. Slowly, he rises and extravagantly stretches his 2-year-old frame, first backward and then forward. He sits up and considers his next move.

In the distance, a resident approaches. It is Mrs. P., who has been living on the dementia unit's third floor for 3 years now. She has long forgotten her family, even though they visit her almost daily. Moderately disheveled after eating her lunch, half of which she now wears on her shirt, Mrs. P. is taking one of her many aimless strolls to nowhere. She glides toward Oscar, pushing her walker and muttering to herself with complete disregard for her surroundings. Perturbed, Oscar watches her carefully and, as she walks by, lets out a gentle hiss, a rattlesnake-like warning that says "leave me alone." She passes him without a glance and continues down the hallway. Oscar is relieved. It is not yet Mrs. P.'s time, and he wants nothing to do with her.

Oscar jumps down off the desk, relieved to be once more alone and in control of his domain. He takes a few moments to drink from his water bowl and grab a quick bite. Satisfied, he enjoys another stretch and sets out on his rounds. Oscar decides to head down the west wing first, along the way sidestepping Mr. S., who is slumped over a couch in the hallway. With lips slightly pursed, he snores peacefully — perhaps blissfully unaware of where he is now living. Oscar continues down the hallway until he reaches its end and Room 310. The door is closed, so Oscar sits and waits. He has important business here.

Twenty-five minutes later, the door finally opens, and out walks a nurse's aide carrying dirty linens. "Hello, Oscar," she says. "Are you going inside?" Oscar lets her pass, then makes his way into the room, where there are two people. Lying in a corner bed and facing the wall, Mrs. T. is asleep in a fetal position. Her body is thin and wasted from the breast cancer that has been eating away at her organs. She is mildly jaundiced and has not spoken in several days. Sitting next to her is her daughter, who glances up from her novel to warmly greet the visitor. "Hello, Oscar. How are you today?"

Oscar takes no notice of the woman and leaps up onto the bed. He surveys Mrs. T. She is clearly in the terminal phase of illness, and her breathing is labored. Oscar's examination is interrupted by a nurse, who walks in to ask the daughter whether Mrs. T. is uncomfortable and needs more morphine. The daughter shakes her head, and the nurse retreats. Oscar returns to his work. He sniffs the air, gives Mrs. T. one final look, then jumps off the bed and quickly leaves the room. Not today.

Making his way back up the hallway, Oscar arrives at Room 313. The door is open, and he proceeds inside. Mrs. K. is resting peacefully in her bed, her breathing steady but shallow. She is surrounded by photographs of her grandchildren and one from her wedding day. Despite these keepsakes, she is alone. Oscar jumps onto her bed and again sniffs the air. He pauses to consider the situation, and then turns around twice before curling up beside Mrs. K.

One hour passes. Oscar waits. A nurse walks into the room to check on her patient. She pauses to note Oscar's presence. Concerned, she hurriedly leaves the room and returns to her desk. She grabs Mrs. K.'s chart off the medical-records rack and begins to make phone calls.

Within a half hour the family starts to arrive. Chairs are brought into the room, where the relatives begin their vigil. The priest is called to deliver last rites. And still, Oscar has not budged, instead purring and gently nuzzling Mrs. K. A young grandson asks his mother, "What is the cat doing here?" The mother, fighting back tears, tells him, "He is here to help Grandma get to heaven." Thirty minutes later, Mrs. K. takes her last earthly breath. With this, Oscar sits up, looks around, then departs the room so quietly that the grieving family barely notices.

On his way back to the charting area, Oscar passes a plaque mounted on the wall. On it is engraved a commendation from a local hospice agency: "For his compassionate hospice care, this plaque is awarded to Oscar the Cat." Oscar takes a quick drink of water and returns to his desk to curl up for a long rest. His day's work is done. There will be no more deaths today, not in Room 310 or in any other room for that matter. After all, no one dies on the third floor unless Oscar pays a visit and stays awhile.

Note: Since he was adopted by staff members as a kitten, Oscar the Cat has had an uncanny ability to predict when residents are about to die. Thus far, he has presided over the deaths of more than 25 residents on the third floor of Steere House Nursing and

Rehabilitation Center in Providence, Rhode Island. His mere presence at the bedside is viewed by physicians and nursing home staff as an almost absolute indicator of impending death, allowing staff members to adequately notify families. Oscar has also provided companionship to those who would otherwise have died alone. For his work, he is highly regarded by the physicians and staff at Steere House and by the families of the residents whom he serves.

The New England Journal of Medicine, July 20, 2007より

◐ Checking the terms

GLOSSARY

award	[賞などを]与える	in a fetal position	胎児のように丸くなって
be slumped over	〜にぐったりともたれかかる	jaundiced	黄疸にかかった
blissfully	このうえなく幸せに	labored breathing	苦しい呼吸
budge	身動きする	last rites	臨終の儀式
charting area	カルテ記入エリア	make one's way back	帰途に就く
commendation	表彰、称賛	make one's way into	[部屋など]に入る
compassionate	心の優しい、哀れみ深い	mutter	ブツブツつぶやく
dementia	認知症	nursing home	老人ホーム、養護施設
disheveled	[服装・髪などが]乱れた、だらしない	peer	じっと見つめる
earthly	[天上ではなく]この世の	perturbed	動揺して、不安がって
engrave	[文字を]刻む	plaque	飾り額
glide	滑るように動く		
hallway	廊下		

retreat	退く、退出する	terminal phase	末期
round	[定められたコースの] 巡回、回診	vigil	徹夜の看病
set out on	～に出発する	walker	歩行器(具)
sidestep	よける、回避する	wasted	衰えた、やつれた
snore	いびきをかく	west/east wing	西(東)棟
take one's last breath	息をひきとる		

Learning the vocabulary

A) 次のリストの単語およびフレーズから最も適当なものを選び、必要なら形を変えて、1～10のセンテンスを完成させましょう。

Here are some words and phrases that are useful to know. Choose the best word or phrase to complete each sentence below with the correct form.

award	labored breathing	take one's last breath
dementia	make one's way into	waste
disheveled	set out on	
jaundiced	slumped over	

1. She (1)_____ after a long battle with leukemia.

2. That woman in her 80s suffers from (2)_____ .

3. He was (3)_____ the Arts Festival Grand Prize.

4. The young man (4)_____ a round-the-world voyage in a sailing boat.

5. Excess bilirubin in a newborn causes the yellowish or (5)_____ color of the skin and eyes.

6. The computer virus (6)_____ the various computers in the company network.

7. The drunken man was (7)_____ the steering wheel of a vehicle stopped in the middle of a road.

8. The child suffers from a disease called asthma, which is marked by attacks of (8)_____ .

9. The (9)_____ man was wearing dirty clothes and had long tangled hair.

10. He had (10)_____ away due to his illness.

B) テキスト中で、次の1～6の猫の動作は英語でどのように表されていますか？　A～Fの中から適切な表現を見つけて線で結びましょう。

How are the cat's movements expressed in the text? Match the Japanese and English phrases.

1 シューと小さく音を立てる	・	・ **A**	leaps up onto ~.
2 まるくなる	・	・ **B**	extravagantly stretches the frame, first backward and then forward.
3 クンクン臭いを嗅ぐ	・	・ **C**	purrs and gently nuzzles
4 前後に大きく伸びをする	・	・ **D**	curls up
5 ゴロゴロと喉を鳴らし、鼻をすり寄せる	・	・ **E**	sniffs the air
6 ぴょんと跳躍して～に飛び乗る	・	・ **F**	lets out a gentle hiss

Understanding the material

オスカーが"診察"した入所者について、名前、"診察"場所、その日の入所者のようす、オスカーの行動と診断, 入所者の家族と職員のようすについて、テキストを参照しながら次の表を完成させましょう。

Compare the following table with information on the residents that Oscar visited.

入所者名 Who?	診察場所 Where?	その日の入所者の様子 Resident's condition	オスカーの行動と診断 (Dying/Not Dying) Oscar's actions and diagnosis	家族と職員の様子・行動 Actions of family and staff
_____ (living in the dementia unit for 3 years)	Charting area	• Gets her shirt dirty with lunch • Walks aimlessly • _____ a walker • _____ to herself • _____ the surroundings completely	• _____ her carefully • Lets out a hiss, meaning "_____" [Dying/Not Dying]	
_____	In the West Wing	• _____ a couch • _____ peacefully • _____ where he is now living	• Sidesteps Mr. S. • Continues down the hallway [Dying/Not Dying]	
_____ (in the terminal phase of breast cancer)	Room ____	• _____ in a fetal position • Mildly _____ • Labored breathing	• Sits and waits for 25 minutes until the door opens • _____ into the room • _____ onto the bed • Surveys her • His examination interrupted by a nurse • Returns to his work • _____ the air • _____ the bed • _____ the room [Dying/Not Dying]	• A nurse's aide walks out • Mrs. T.'s daughter _____ • A nurse _____, talks to the daughter to confirm that Mrs. T does not need more _____, and walks out

| _____ Room ____ | • _____ peacefully in her bed
• Her breathing _____ but _____
• Alone, surrounded by _____ of her family
• _____ 30 minutes after her family's arrival | • Proceeds inside
• _____ onto her bed
• _____ the air
• _____ the situation
• _____ twice
• _____ beside her
• Waits for an hour
• _____ nuzzles Mrs. K.
• Sits up, looks around, and _____
• _____ to his desk to _____ for a long rest
[Dying/Not Dying] | • A nurse walks into the room; pauses to _____; and hurriedly _____
• A nurse begins to _____
• Within a half hour, the family _____ _____; and _____
• The priest is called to _____ |

Trying out the genre

A) Understanding the material の表に書き込まれた情報を用いて、この日 Mrs. K に起こったことを要約してみましょう。出来事は、時間に沿って起こった順に記述しましょう。

Use the information for Mrs. K in the table of the above section and summarize what happened to Mrs. K in the order in which the events occurred.

B) このテキストの著者 (老人科の医師) は、一連の出来事に対する著者自身の考えを述べないことで、それを読者に委ねるという手法をとっています。著者は読者に何を考えてほしかったのでしょうか？　オスカーはわたしたちに何を教えてくれていますか？　いろいろな意見を出しあってみてください。

This text was written by a gerontologist describing the actions of a cat living in a nursing home. The author does not specifically state his feelings but is sending out a message to the readers. What do you think it might be? Discuss various possibilities.

📋 Applying what you learned

A) The New England Journal of Medicine は、誌面の大部分が投稿記事で構成されています。このテキストはPerspective articleという記事ですが、ほかにどんな種類の投稿記事があるかをこの雑誌の投稿規定のウェブページで調べてみましょう。

The New England Journal of Medicine carries many submitted articles. The Perspective article presented here is one of several types that can be submitted. Check the instructions to authors for NEJM to find what other types of articles can be submitted.

http://www.nejm.org/page/author-center/article-types

B) 上記の投稿規定のページによるとPerspective articleについては、次のように指示しています。
The instructions for authors describe the Perspective article as follows:

Perspective articles cover a wide variety of topics of current interest in health care, medicine, and the intersection between medicine and society.

1）NEJMのPerspectiveを集めたウェブページ
（http://www.nejm.org/browse?category=perspective）を見て、どのようなトピックが選ばれているかを調べましょう。
Check the NEJM Perspective article website and identify the topics presented.

2）もし、この雑誌にPerspective articleという種類の記事を投稿するとすれば、どのようなトピックで記事を書いてみたいか話しあってみましょう。
If you were to write a Perspective article for submission to NEJM, what topic would you choose to write about?

Relaxing a bit

オープンアクセスポリシー

　オープンアクセスとは、査読付き学術雑誌に掲載された論文を、インターネット上で誰もが無料で閲覧できる状態にしておくことを指します。インターネットの普及を背景にして、近年広まり、結実した運動です。法制化の動きも進んでおり、2007年末にはアメリカ合衆国で、アメリカ国立衛生研究所 (NIH) から予算を受けて行った研究の成果は、発表後一年以内に公衆が無料でアクセスできる状態にしなければならない、ということが法律で義務化されました。New England Journal of Medicineの記事は、発行より6カ月遅れでオンラインアクセスすることができます。後発開発途上国には、この6カ月の遅延は適用されず、個人利用に限り発行と同時に無料閲覧ができます。

著者紹介

野口 ジュディー（Ph.D.）
2001年 バーミンガム大学大学院英語研究科修了
現　在 神戸学院大学　名誉教授
　　　　大阪大学大学院工学研究科　非常勤講師
　　　　大阪大学大学院医学系研究科　非常勤講師
　　　　神戸大学大学院工学研究科　非常勤講師
　　　　神戸大学大学院保健学研究科　非常勤講師

神前 陽子（Ed.D.）
2006年 テンプル大学大学院英語教授法研究科修了
現　在 武庫川女子大学薬学部　非常勤講師
　　　　大阪医科薬科大学　非常勤講師
　　　　神戸大学大学院理学研究科　非常勤講師
　　　　テンプル大学応用言語学博士課程　非常勤講師

スミス 朋子（Ph.D.）
2005年 カリフォルニア大学バークレー校大学院言語学研究科修了
現　在 大阪医科薬科大学薬学部　教授

天ヶ瀬 葉子（Ph.D.）
2002年 ケンブリッジ大学大学院生物学研究科薬理学専攻修了
現　在 大阪医科薬科大学薬学部　准教授
　　　　京都薬科大学　非常勤講師

NDC491　　103p　　26cm

はじめての薬学英語

2013年3月27日　第 1 刷発行
2024年3月 8日　第13刷発行

著　者　野口ジュディー・神前陽子・スミス朋子・天ヶ瀬葉子
発行者　森田浩章
発行所　株式会社　講談社
　　　　〒112-8001　東京都文京区音羽2-12-21
　　　　　販　売　(03) 5395-4415
　　　　　業　務　(03) 5395-3615
編　集　株式会社　講談社サイエンティフィク
　　　　代表　堀越俊一
　　　　〒162-0825　東京都新宿区神楽坂2-14　ノービィビル
　　　　　編　集　(03) 3235-3701
DTP　　株式会社エヌ・オフィス
印刷所　株式会社平河工業社
製本所　株式会社国宝社

落丁本・乱丁本は購入書店名を明記のうえ，講談社業務宛にお送りください．送料小社負担にてお取替えします．なお，この本の内容についてのお問い合わせは，講談社サイエンティフィク宛にお願いいたします．価格はカバーに表示してあります．

© J. Noguchi, Y. Kozaki, T. Smith and Y. Amagase, 2013

本書のコピー，スキャン，デジタル化等の無断複製は著作権法上での例外を除き禁じられています．本書を代行業者等の第三者に依頼してスキャンやデジタル化することはたとえ個人や家庭内の利用でも著作権法違反です．

[JCOPY] 〈（社）出版者著作権管理機構　委託出版物〉

複写される場合は，その都度事前に（社）出版者著作権管理機構（電話 03-5244-5088, FAX 03-5244-5089, e-mail: info@jcopy.or.jp）の許諾を得てください．

Printed in Japan

ISBN978-4-06-155619-5